Think Yourself Skinny

Change Your Mind & Change Your Life

[MARLON J. DUGAR]

negligence, personal injury, criminal intent, or under any other cause of action.

You agree to accept all risks of using the information presented inside this book.

You agree that by continuing to read this book, where appropriate and/or necessary, you shall consult a professional (including but not limited to your doctor, attorney, or financial advisor or such other advisor as needed) before using any of the suggested remedies, techniques, or information in this book.

Table of Contents

Introduction

Congratulations are in order! The reason I say that is because the fact that you have chosen to change the way you have been thinking about yourself, and what you are capable of, deserves a bit of praise. You have just put yourself in the driver's seat of a brand-new future that will reward you over and over.

You are about to indulge in a system that I've prepared for those of us that were not born with perfect physiques and had struggled to find something that works in aiding us in our goal of losing the weight and gaining the confidence!

If you are like me, you've probably spent 100's if not 1000's of dollars on those celebrity diet programs, or those crazy fitness DVDs only to find out that none of the people on the DVD or that promote the program look ANYTHING like you!! Isn't that strange how we look at this and believe that these people have any clue about the real struggle millions of people face year after year to be free from the feeling of worthlessness and insecurity because of the excess weight? I've been there.

I weighed a staggering 300+ pounds (around 340lbs) and struggled many days to love the person I saw in the mirror. I'd bought programs in the past that promised crazy results, only to find out that these programs were built and designed for people already in shape. So needless to say, I never had the motivation to continue any of them. My real motivation came in 2017 when I came dangerously close to dying of a heart attack. I had to be admitted to the hospital for treatment. I have to admit to you, I WAS TERRIFIED. Earlier that day I felt normal, and later that day I was on my death bed. Need-less to say that put me in a different mode of thinking. I started to research many of the popular diets and found that although they were similar, the information they gave contradicted other so-called top diet programs. After extensive research I concluded that there is NOT a one size fits all diet for every person in the world. Each is made differently, shaped differently, and what I've found out to be the most important thing is, THINK DIFFERENTLY!

In this system, you will see that I have put together a program that uniquely adapts to the need of the individual. You will be able to pick the way you want to look, and it all starts with the way you THINK. I have a Step-By-Step- Guide on what you need to do and when starting you from day one. But, before we dive in, I'd like to debunk some things you've probably heard before that are not true and might be the cause of your failed success at Weight Loss.

In this book, I show you how to ditch the carbs and excess pounds without giving up flavor or feeling like you're starving. When you switch from burning glucose as your primary fuel—the natural result of a high-carb diet—to burning fat instead, you will lose weight, feel satisfied, and finally be in control of what you eat. It is such an empowering feeling!

My approach is flexible and takes into consideration that life happens. It took me 9months and it will be appropriate for you to follow the guidance in the whole book. Unlike other diets that require you to start all over again if you deviate by even a crumb, this program rejects the all-or-nothing approach. If you exceed your carbs one day, let it go and move on to the next day. With dedication you will lose weight, change your relationship with food, and change your life!

Weight loss is the weight that you lose when your body undergoes a process of what experts classify as a caloric deficiency. This can be achieved either by boosting your calories requirement through the building of muscle mass while keeping your intake constant or via calorie restriction in the form of a diet where your daily calorie intake is designed to be lesser than your daily requirement.

When your body finds itself in a state where calories input is lesser than what it needs to daily function, it will seek to get energy from stores of energy within your body. Most of the time these would be from the stores of glucose found in the liver as well as from your muscle. The other major energy store found in our body would be the fats that we carry on our frame. This is where the tricky part comes in. If your body isn't conditioned for burning fats, it will quickly use up the glucose stores, and that is when the feeling of hunger will come into potentially derail you from your weight loss mission.

Chapter 1: My guide to weight loss

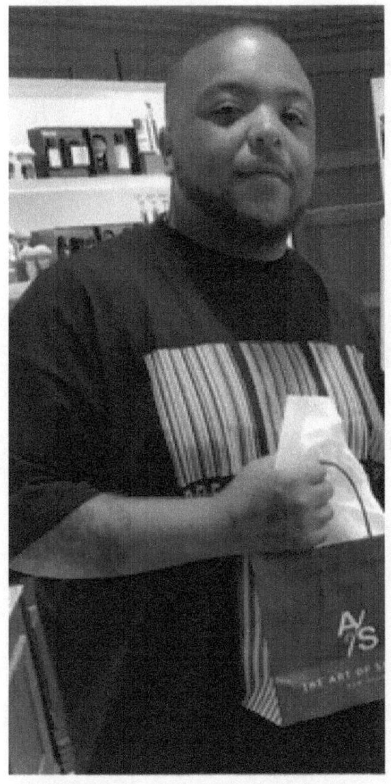

You Can Shrink Your Stomach?

What? This is some of the foolishness that I'm talking about that is out there! In short, NO! You can't shrink your stomach! This is impossible, seeing that your stomach is made much like a rubber band. Try to shrink a rubber band, go ahead I'll wait. That can't happen, but what can happen is, you CAN stretch your stomach like a rubber band. Your mind controls even the stretching of your stomach, but we'll talk more about that in the system.

• If You Don't Eat Your Body Will Store Fat?

This topic is controversial because it is only partially correct. Your body doesn't control what happens to it, your BRAIN does. If I tell my body we are going to exercise today, regardless if I've eaten or not; my body will get up and exercise. Regardless if there is stored fat or not, my body will be forced to use whatever energy reserves it has to do the exercise I command it to. Your body will adjust to what YOU say. Remember, YOU are in control.

• You Can TARGET Weight Loss?

Really? If this were true, I would lose weight in my target area and not in others. How long have you "targeted" weight loss in a particular area, and found that you may have lost weight, but that "targeted" area was just overworked and strained. When a person starts to lose weight, they lose all over their body. You might lose in your thighs first, or in your hands, maybe even under your feet.

Chapter 2: Nutrition and Weight Loss

Almost 70-80% of effective weight loss plans rely on diet alone which proves that certain amounts of food and the kinds of nutrients you put in your body may be your single most effective way of dropping the pounds. Nutrition weight loss takes into consideration more than just supplementing your diet with multi-vitamins. It includes portion sizes when you eat certain foods and the kinds of foods you should eat for specific results.

If you research various strategies to lose weight, you will find thousands of different quick fix programs available today. Most of these programs offer a few essentials of legitimate weight loss information, but many times they miss the overall goal. Weight loss is more about a healthy lifestyle then it is a 3-week quick weight loss program that is sure to fail in a few months. As far as nutrition is concerned, there are a few factors you need to consider including calories, carbohydrates, fats, sugars, proteins and more. Choosing a nutritional weight loss program is intended to maximize the benefits of losing pounds through the best combination of nutrients.

One of the first things to change when trying to implement a nutrition weight loss program is the size of your meals. The basic daily caloric intake is 2000 calories, but this is variable depending on the size of the person. If you are a larger individual, your caloric intake may require up to 2500 calories. You should see a nutritionist or dietitian to get a good idea of your individual needs. Other than that, you should be careful to watch your portion sizes in general.

Secondly, eat more frequently, but lesser amounts. Your brain takes about 15 to 20 minutes to sense that your stomach is full, so try slowing down as you eat so a to allow time for your brain to signal to your hunger needs that you are full.

Third, commit to eating the right foods at the right times. In the mornings, you should avoid foods such as egg whites and some whole grain toast. This could be complemented with low-fat yogurt or a fruit of some kind. If you are a cereal lover, then stay away from the sugary cereals and stick with whole grains as well as fibrous cereals. The first half of your day should be the time you should consume the sweets that are in fruits and other cereals. During the PM hours stay away from starches and sugar. You should eat a lot of protein and green vegetables. For snacks, try eating carrots or celery with peanut butter.

Following these simple tips can help you get into shape quicker than ever before and will develop in you a healthier overall lifestyle. Overall, pick healthy versions of the foods you love. Also, any good nutrition and weight loss program can provide you with more extensive guidance and menu suggestions for a fully managed system.

Chapter 3: Weight Loss Principles

To help with the process of losing the unwelcome weight from your body, here are some of the more common principles which are good to base your weight loss strategies on.

Keep hunger at bay – Many folks start off on dieting to lose their excess weight and attempt to get healthy, but quite a number fail and fall by the wayside. In the end, these folks are forced to resort to medications and drugs to suppress the symptoms and conditions that accompany obesity. It is not a pretty sight, and it sometimes is quite depressing to see people consign themselves to such a fate when more efficient and healthier solutions are just around the corner.

They may have started off strong and seen results after some time, but invariably, the one thing that always put paid to these efforts would be the feeling of hunger that many of these diets entail. Take a plain calorie restriction diet plan for example, if your daily requirement works out to be about 1,750 calories, just polishing off a bagel for a snack would set you back by 250 calories. That is like one-seventh of your total requirement. Imagine eating seven bagels for the whole day, would that be enough?

The trick, of course, is to get onto a diet and lifestyle change where you can feel full and keep the hunger pangs at bay and yet get your body to lose weight. Know of any diet that does just that?

Be sustainable – There are many ways to lose weight, that is for sure. Getting on the latest fad diet, juicing, fasting, going the vegan way. I have to say as a matter of the fact that I hold all these methodologies in high esteem and it is my opinion that each one of them has their benefits for the human body.

Fasting, for example, is a good way to let the body rebalance itself and to get rid of toxins that have built up over time. One of the side effects of fasting would be a loss of body weight. However, you would not expect a person to fast for a lifetime, without any consumption of food. For any method of efficient weight loss, it must be sustainable in practice to allow for continued shedding of the excess pounds and to prevent the dreaded bounce back in weight that has plagued so many.

One of the benchmarks of sustainability for diets would be the ease of implementing it in everyday life. Imagine if you are on a diet that requires you to eat six to seven small meals a day, you would have to pack for those meals and find the time to consume them during the workday.

Exercise – Regarded as one of the main pillars for weight loss, exercise, especially strength training, can help to build muscles that burn more calories, not to mention getting you that ripped figure. Yes, it was always good to dream that there was some magic pill in the market that could get you whipped into shape without any effort, but alas, it remains a dream.

Strength training, done through weights at home or by hitting the gym is one of the surest ways that weight can be lost. Most of the time, it would be advisable to have a schedule for the days that you're going to workout, so that you can concentrate on specific muscle groups. This targeted training helps to speed muscle development, leading to higher calorie usage and hence weight loss.

There will be loads of resources online on how to work out a proper strength training routine. The more important thing is to have the discipline to keep plugging at it until you see or feel the results. It will be worth it.

Ketogenic Diet and Weight Loss

Having touched on what weight loss was and the common principles behind it, let us now look at how the ketogenic diet can become one of your staunchest allies in the battle of the bulge.

Being mindful of hunger – As we said earlier, keeping hunger pangs at bay is one of the most important ways to ensure your weight loss regime is on track. The keto diet does this precisely by encouraging the consumption of fats, which by nature is more satiating and gives you the feeling of fulfillment and hence stops those frequent trips to the kitchen pantry for more food.

The other spiffy thing about going on the keto diet is the resultant leveling of your insulin levels. Insulin is known to induce the feeling of hunger and when ketosis kicks in, you no longer have those roller coaster ups and downs that are associated with the consumption of carbs and with that stability means your hunger pangs are held largely at bay due to the reduction of insulin produced by your body.

Now, you will eat when your body truly feels hunger, and that is quite liberating. Not to mention that because of this removal of hunger pangs from the overall equation, your weight loss journey will become much, much simpler.

Quicker recovery from exercise – While we engage in strength training in our bid to lose weight and get in shape, our bodies need time to recover from the physical activity. Practitioners of the keto diet will find that their recovery time will be somewhat quicker than others.

The reduction of carbohydrates to be replaced by fats is one of the main reasons why overall body inflammation levels will come down. Once inflammation is down, your muscles tend to recover faster from fatigue, and this allows you to put in more sessions due to the shortened recovery period. With the more stable energy levels achieved due to fewer fluctuations in the blood sugar levels, again due to the diet switch, this then allows you to work out without feeling faintish or light-headed, typical symptoms of hypoglycemia or just simple lack of glucose in the bloodstream. Because you are burning fats and producing ketones as a more stable energy source!

More motivation from quicker results – Quick question, which would you prefer, a weight loss method that requires you to toil consistently at it for up to six months a pop, and having a loss of four or five pounds to show for it, or the ketogenic diet that can see weight loss come in the range of twenty to thirty pounds within six to seven weeks?

If you are like me, then the choice would be the latter. Quicker results, especially in the area of weight loss, is almost always going to be a welcome morale booster. When you see how much weight you have lost within those short weeks, it gives you that confidence that this method works, and you gain that conviction and strength to keep going.

What happens here when you transit over to the keto diet is the fact that you have lowered insulin levels. Heightened insulin tells our kidneys to retain more salt and water, so when the insulin levels decrease, we have consequently lesser salt and water retention. This leads to a quick decrease in the number on the weighing scales, but more importantly, the keto diet also provides for a sustained drive in the loss of body weight through the burning of fat stores.

Chapter 4: Detox for weight loss

Most of your daily detox efforts to eliminate fungus, bacteria, and cleanse the liver of toxins will assist you in your weight loss efforts. Most often the cause of excess weight is that the body is full of excess stored wastes and toxins, as soon as you remove those in the mentioned protocols you most likely will have lost all the weight you needed to. When the stomach and digestive system are clogged, food cannot be properly absorbed. This puts the body in a constant state of starvation, requiring you to eat more and more. This is exacerbated by traditional weight-loss diets. The answer is to clean out the waste from the body, so you can obtain nutrition and energy from the foods you eat, and to learn how to transition to a diet of live and energy-giving foods that cleanse, and do not clog you. Fruits and vegetables are full of fiber and are very cleansing to the digestive tract, therefore you do not need to be restrictive about your diet as the more you eat the more you cleanse. Worldwide research shows being overweight is frequently linked to insulin resistance (especially due to a diet high in refined carbohydrates). A healthy metabolism is essential to your detoxification system in keeping your body clean and free of bacteria. In addition to having a well-balanced diet, and leading an active lifestyle, there are certain natural herbs and spices that can also be extremely helpful in stimulating your body to detox and burn fat. Antioxidants also boost the metabolism therefore any food or supplement that is rich in antioxidants may be beneficial for weight loss. Here is a program with specific foods and herbs that can help target and break down fatty tissue.

Herbs for weight loss

Hawthorn

The hawthorn berry helps to metabolize, stagnant undigested food in the stomach.

Reduces blood fat and improves circulation. Hawthorn berry helps with stagnant, undigested food accumulated in the stomach, they also stimulate the adrenal glands and improve thyroid function. Do you love sweets and can't seem to get enough of it? If sugar is the one that gets you down in your weight loss and detox plans, try Gymnema Sylvestre. You wouldn't believe that there really is a miracle pill to take against food cravings.

Gymnema Sylvestre

It was used as far back as 2,000 years ago in India for diabetes, and obesity. If taken with a meal, the gymnema molecules, similar to glucose, fill the taste receptors on the tongue preventing the taste buds from being activated by real sugar. It also inhibits the intestine from absorbing sugar from the food you eat.

Lemon

Personally, during my weight loss journey, I used Laci LE BEAU, SUPER DIETER'S TEA" Lemon Mint Flavor. Lemon- is a number one weight loss food due to its cleansing and detoxifying abilities. Take in the morning with warm water and salt to cleanse your liver and digestive system. Lemon is also very beneficial for improving the function of the lymphatic system.

Salt flush and coffee enema cleanse

Mix 1 t. of sea salt into 16 oz of warm water, drink first thing in the morning. This is the easiest intestinal cleanse you can possibly do. It cleanses the entire digestive tract, not just the colon. The saltwater will pass through your intestines and you should be able to flush your entire digestive tract within an hour or two. If no movement occurs, it may mean the person is salt deficient and may need more than one flush to get good results.

Lie on your right side for 30 minutes this is to ensure that the water goes straight into the small intestines on the lower right side of the stomach. The muscle contractions in the small intestines will then carry the water down and flush everything out on its way. You can do this once a week or once a month for before doing a coffee enema to clear everything out of the digestive tract. It can also be done daily for no more than two weeks. Although water retention is very rare, if it does occur, discontinue using the flush for a few days and use diuretic and kidney cleansing herbs such as dandelion and horsetail.

Chapter 5: Food Guide for Weight loss

Food is a word that when mentioned, everybody views it as something worth consumption. But do we ever stop to think whether all foods are suitable for us? Do we also take caution on how much food we ought to take? There are distinct types of foods such as carbohydrates, proteins, vitamins, minerals, and water. Well, they are all meant for the good of our bodies, but most importantly, we must take note of how much of these foods we consume.

Do you want to lose weight? You do not have to stop eating to achieve the same. Below are some guidelines on how to manage your weight while still attending to your stomach needs.

Carbohydrates

EAT LESS CARBS

I found that food is the only means that could propel me to lose weight and keep healthy by ensuring proper feeding habits. That's why I wanted to present these three shreds of evidence that explain the benefit of low carbohydrate diet. The carbohydrate diets are so effective that they are prescribed to the overweight people.

Carbohydrate consumption in a day

You're not safe to consume too much or not enough carbohydrates. To lose weight, reducing the intake of carbs is core. Eating fewer carbs reduces your appetite and automatically necessitates weight loss even without calorie restriction.

Optimum carbohydrate intake depends on age, gender, activity levels, body composition, metabolic health and food culture.

For people who are lean or simply trying to maintain their weight and stay healthy, their carbohydrate intake should range between 100-150 grams per day

To understand the required daily carb intake, it's advisable to comprehend several types of carbohydrates.

Best Vitamins

Vitamins could be used as a perfect way to keep a healthy body with an ideal weight. Some of these vitamins are discussed below:

(a) Vitamin B12

Vitamin B12 soluble in water and is usually essential in ensuring proper usage of calories in the body as well as red blood cell creation. This vitamin is found in some animal proteins such as beef, chicken, and fish. Vitamin B12 is necessary for giving the body the required energy which results to more psyche to exercise and eventually weight loss.

(b) Fiber

So here is another vitamin that most of us don't pay attention to. Research has shown that taking high amounts of fiber results to reduced appetite which then means fewer calories are taken in. A person who consumes large amounts of fiber stands a chance to improve his or her digestion and an excellent opportunity to lose weight without having to take in any pills.

(c) Chromium

Chromium is a mineral that is necessary for sugar metabolism as well as aiding to keep proper fat levels. People who consume chromium have been observed to record high levels of weight loss.

APPROPRIATE VITAMIN AND MINERAL INTAKE

So, you want to lose weight healthily? Then mind the vitamin and mineral quantities consumed. Vitamins are in some way meant to supplement the food you take. You, therefore, should be careful not to make them your primary food. Excess consumption of vitamins and minerals results to over-accumulation in the body especially for the ones that are soluble in fats. Precaution must be taken since too much of it is harmful, and nobody eats to cause harm to their body.

WATER

If you want to be healthy with the best weight possible, then I have what you need; water. Being free from calories, water is the drink to take most often. One should take at least 5 liters of water per day.

WATER FOR WEIGHT LOSS

Have you ever realized that you eat less when you drink water before taking your meals? If you have not realized that, then it is high time you tried that out. Drinking a lot of water increases the amount of fluids in your body yet you can still use it for appetite loss. That means you will be losing weight but boosting fluid levels in your body. Good strategy, isn't it?

HOW MUCH WATER FOR FIT WEIGHT LOSS

You must be thinking that no matter the amount of water taken, it does not matter? Well, that is not the case. Two glasses of water before every meal is enough to reduce appetite. Remember, I am not asking you to suppress your appetite completely. You need to remain healthy, and so you must take appropriate amounts of food. Excessive water becomes a burden to the kidney to push it all out of the body resulting to waterlogging in the blood. Am sure you do not want that.

Tips to eat Carbs without stoking much fat

Every time you eat carbohydrates with a high glycemic index, there is a significant amount of sugar that comes in your blood. When you have a high blood sugar your survival is at stake, so your body releases a large amount of insulin to lower your rates as soon as possible.

Therefore, you should never eat sugar outside dining. You can eat your carbs with a source of fat, protein or fibrous vegetables that will slow their digestion and regulate the release of sugar into your bloodstream. Also, you can eat only low glycemic foods, which are broken down and digested slowly.

By doing this, you will enjoy the most of your carbohydrates as an energy source and will limit fat storage.

Avoid Carbs that are processed as fat

When your body energy is excess, and your glycogen stores (muscles and liver) are full, the surplus carbohydrates you eat is turned into fat. The ideal time to consume your carbs is in the morning and around your workouts.

When to eat your Carbs

To avoid running out of carbohydrates or ruin your body and your health because of them, I will now tell you when to eat your carbs. Most people store fat when they eat carbohydrates because they deplete the wrong time. If you consume your carbohydrates at specific times slammed on your lifestyle, you will not have to worry about taking fat.

Proteins

Proteins are foods that when taken, they help in building the body as well as repairing the body tissues. If you want to have a proper looking body, the protein is your answer. They include legumes, beef, chicken, and milk. Am sure you can access at least a few of these foods. So how do proteins aid in weight loss?

Eat Large amounts of Protein

High amounts of proteins are healthy when taken for bodybuilding and for reducing weight. When you consume large quantities of proteins, the rate of metabolism is equally high. This is paramount in ensuring reduction of appetite and therefore regulating weight-related hormones. What proteins do to reduce weight is reduce your appetite so eventually your calories levels drop automatically.

Making right Protein Choices

I just took you through the necessity of high proteins for weight loss. However, you must not forget that there is a limit beyond which when proteins are considered, they become detrimental to your health. Remember our focus is attaining a healthy body with reduced weight; or else you focus on reducing weight and forget that your body ought to remain healthy.

Proteins that are best for your health

You are already aware that you should not take extreme levels of proteins. It is, therefore, important to know what proteins are best when taken and which ones should be avoided.

Animal proteins such as beef, chicken, and fish are best when taken since they provide you with all amino acids. This is not to say plant proteins are not advisable. I am just stating that, if you need high levels of Amino acids all at once, and then feed on animal proteins since plant proteins provide reduced levels of Amino acids. Most importantly, we must be careful with processed proteins since they consist, for instance, embedded salts that could result in increased blood pressure levels. Therefore, know what proteins to consume, in what amounts to ensure you keep your goal of weight loss while remaining healthy in check.

Vitamins and Minerals

Vitamins and minerals are compounds that are organic and are usually consumed in small amounts because the body cannot synthesize them. They facilitate proper functioning of the body after consumption of the other major food components. Examples of foods that provide the body with vitamins and minerals are; carrots, tropical fruits, dark leafy greens, calcium, chromium, and squash potatoes.

Chapter 6: Exercise Benefits

Exercise is proven to be one of the best ways to improve your physical and mental health. People from various age groups can exercise to lose weight. You don't even have to be a fitness fanatic to enjoy the benefits of a good workout. Fortunately, there are easy and fun activities to help you live a healthier and happier life.

Benefits of Exercise:

-Release anxiety and stress

Aerobic exercise releases relaxing hormones which relieves stress. It also promotes a better well-being.

-More brainpower

Exercise promotes the development of brain cells and can help you concentrate better.

-Boosting energy

Exercising several times per week can give you more energy and improve your endurance. When your heart and lungs work efficiently, you will have more energy to complete your daily tasks.

-Weight loss

Exercise is proven to reduce the chances of weight gain. Fortunately, you don't have to spend too much time to get the full benefits.

-Promotes sleep

Regular exercise can help people fall asleep faster but does not exercise too close to your bedtime or you will feel too energized to fall asleep.

Chapter 7: Intermittent fasting

It involves alternating you're eating pattern between periods of fasting (consuming only water) and non-fasting (eating). The eating times can be highly variable and extend over several days. Some of the longer non-eating periods include a 36-hour fast followed by 12 hours of eating (usually broken into 3 meals about 3-4 hours apart) Most intermittent fasting diets extend over a 24-hour period, allowing the person to stay consistent from day to day. The more aggressive of these day-long fasts limit a person to 4 hours of eating (usually at night). The most widely accepted fasting regimen involves an 8-hour window for eating.

Intermittent fasting has been studied extensively on both animals and humans. Unless the fast was extended beyond 36 hours, no negative effects were observed in the test subjects (other than mild to moderate hunger pains). Intermittent fasting has been shown to decrease body fat, stabilize blood sugars, and increase muscle response.

How does it work? It all revolves around the hormone insulin. Your body releases insulin whenever you consume food (more so for foods high in carbohydrates). The insulin stimulates the absorption of nutrients (mostly glucose) into your fat and muscle tissue. Since most of the time, the muscle cells are not energy deprived, excess nutrients after meals are stored in your fat tissue (glucose is also stored as glycogen in your liver). It takes about 3 hours after meal times before your body's insulin level drops to pre-meal levels. At the lower insulin concentrations, your liver and fat tissue release the stored glucose and fatty acids into your bloodstream for energy. By extending the time between meals, you increase the length of this catabolic state when your body burns off fat.

Were you told to eat 5-6 small meals each day? Frequent meal consumption hinders the body's fat-burning process. Under a similar diet, a person using an intermittent fasting approach will attain a lower body fat percentage than the frequent eater. Keep in mind, however, that the quality of your diet is more important than the timing. Intermittent fasting is not an excuse for binging on junk food later at night. You still need to eat clean. Furthermore, you will want to increase your protein consumption when on a fasting diet. Protein is the best macronutrient regarding satiety, meaning that calorie-for-calorie, protein will subdue the feeling of hunger for longer than will carbohydrates or fats. Eating a high-protein/low-carb diet is a must, especially on non-workout days.

Chapter 8: Advantages of Intermittent Fasting

1. Encourages Weight Loss

The most profound advantage of intermittent fasting is due to how it boosts your body's capacity to burn fat and help individuals to maintain their weight and build a better physique. Intermittent fasting, in my opinion, is more adaptable that most dieting strategies because it eliminates the factors of you having to track the number of calories per meal.

Intermittent fasting essentially forces your body to exhaust fat it had previously stored for energy, this process then increases the fat burning process which in turn improves weight loss because your body uses sugar (glucose) which is the primary source for our body's energy when you eat, it then stores what is not absorbed in your liver, and muscles as glycogen.

When our body is deprived of a constant glucose supply, it is forced to break down the reserves of glycogen and use it as a source fuel. After which your body will look for a new source of energy (generally your fat cells). These fat cells with then are broken down to help your body produce energy.

2. Assists in Regulating Blood Sugar

When carbohydrates are consumed the body converts it to sugar (glucose) in the bloodstream. Insulin is the hormone responsible for transferring glucose from the bloodstream into cells to be used as an energy source.

When the body suffers from ailments such as diabetes, it fails to produce insulin properly which causes elevated levels of glucose in the bloodstream (diabetes). This then leaves the body suffering from complications such as thirst, frequent urination, and fatigue.

Analysis of intermittent fasting has revealed findings that indicate your body improves from the process as it regulates your blood sugar levels, stopping spikes and crashes.

3.Takes Care of Your Heart

One of the most profound intermittent fasting advantages is the effect it has on the heart. Findings have indicated that the process has correlated with reduced heart disease complications.

A study of the process showcased the vast influence fasting had on factors directly related to heart health. They observed increased levels good HDL cholesterol and a decrease in bad LDL cholesterol and triglyceride levels.

An animal study reviewed in the Nutritional Biochemistry Journal showed that IMF (intermittent fasting) resulted in a spike in adiponectin levels. The protein that aids the processing of sugars is called Adiponectin; They are said to be defensive in preventing cardiac arrest, and heart diseases. One of the studies on rats noticed that the ones who fasted were 66% likelier to survive a heart attack than the ones on a regular diet.

4. Lessens Inflammation Levels

Inflammation is the bodies response to an infection or injury. Chronic inflammation, however, may result in chronic disease.

Researchers have determined that inflammation can be linked to chronic conditions such as obesity, diabetes, heart disease and cancer.

A study of 50 individuals partaking in Ramadan was released in the Nutrition Research journal. The findings indicated that the levels of some inflammation markers in the participants decreased during the fasting. In 2015 a separate study revealed that longer spans of night fasting were directly correlated to decreased markers of inflammation.

It has been noted that more in-depth studies are needed in the area, but the available studies have uncovered enough evidence to determine that intermittent fasting could help with the reduction of inflammation and other chronic diseases.

5. Protects the Brain

intermittent fasting has not only been proven to improve your chances of chronic diseases such as heart disease, diabetes, and obesity. further studies into intermittent fasting has indicated that it could possibly protect the health of your brain

An animal study revealed that intermittent fasting improved cognitive functions and provided protected against changes in memory and learning function when compared to a controlled group.

Additionally, researchers have noted that anti-inflammatory effects of intermittent fasting can enhance your brain functions which can reduce the progress of diseases like Parkinson's, Alzheimer's, and dementia.

6. Reduces Hunger Surges

The hormone responsible for controlling hunger is called Leptin. It is produced when your fat cells signal sends a signal to our body telling it to stop eating. The level of leptin in the body determines hunger. When the levels drop your body feels hunger, and they rise you feel full.

Individuals who are obese usually have higher levels of leptin in their bodies this occurs because the production of this hormone is primary in the body's fat cells. If he body produces an excess amount of leptin, it can make the body resistant to signals that notify the body to stop eating.

A study of 80 individuals whose leptin levels were measured while on intermittent fasting revealed that the hormone levels became lower at night which means they tend to get hungrier at night. This indicates that eating throughout the day and fasting at night could translate to reduced hunger urges leading to further weight loss.

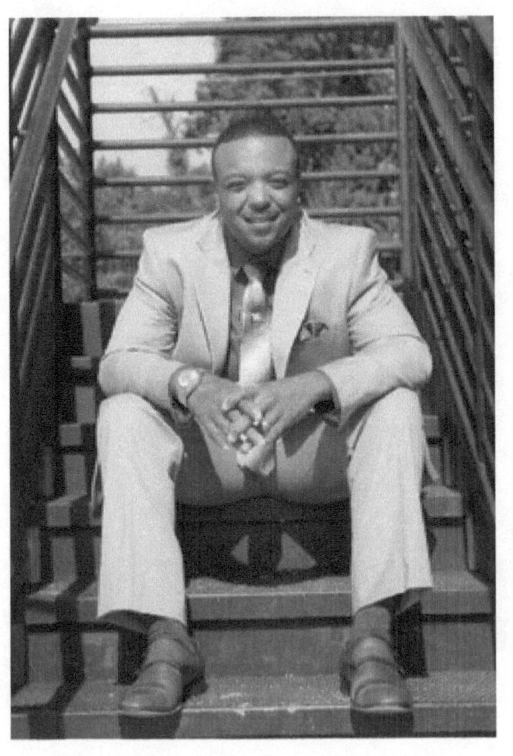

Chapter 9: Breakfast Recipes

Spinach and Swiss Quiche

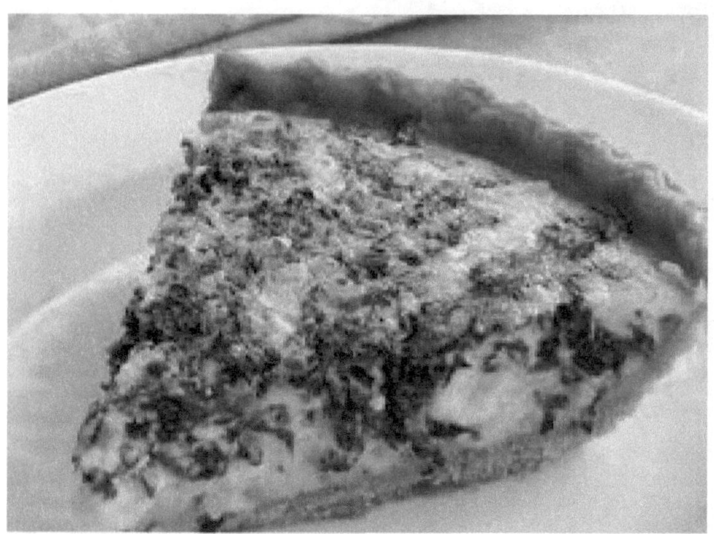

Prep time: 19 minutes

Cook time: 29 minutes

Serves: 4

Ingredients

- 2 tablespoon butter

- 6 oz. frozen chopped spinach, drained and thawed

- 1 cup cream

- 1 cup hand-shredded swiss cheese or hand-shredded cheese

- ¼ tablespoon salt

- 1 diced white onion

- 4 eggs

- ⅛ tablespoon nutmeg

- ¼ tablespoon black pepper, ground

Directions

1. Heat the oven to 350 degrees.

2. Then spray a pie pan with your choice of cooking spray. Spray liberally as eggs may stick.

3. Cook onions in butter till glassy, then add the spinach and simmer until the water is gone.

4. Mix all the ingredients in a bowl, including the spices.

5. Pour into the pie pan.

6. Bake for 29 minutes.

7. Cool for 9 minutes and cut into quarters.

8. Wrap a cooled slice of quiche in saran wrap, then place in a zip-lock bag. Microwave for 1 minute in two 30-second bursts.

Nutritional Value: Calories: 417, Total Fat: 37g, Protein: 15g, Total Carbs: 4g, Dietary Fiber: 1.5g, Sugar: 0g, Sodium: 209mg

Sausage Egg Muffins

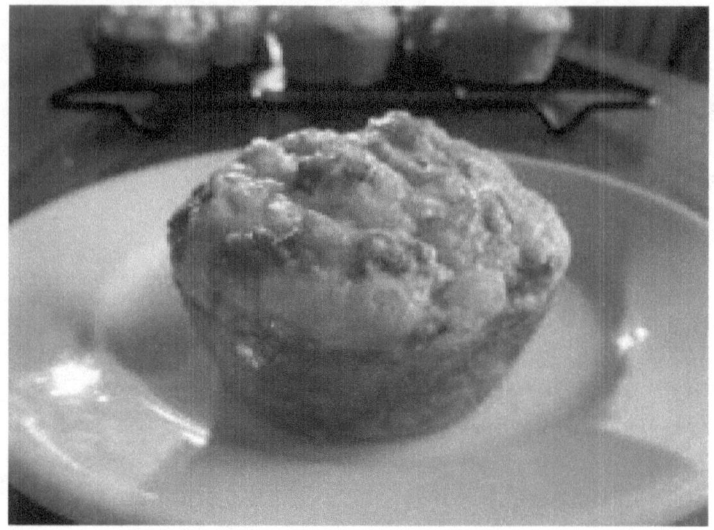

Prep time: 10minutes

Cook time: 29 minutes

Serves: 12

Ingredients

- 12 oz. cooked sausage crumbles

- 12 eggs

- ¼ cup milk

- 2 cups cheddar cheese, sharp, hand-shredded

- ¼ tablespoon black pepper or chili pepper

Directions

1. Mix all the ingredients.

2. Pour into 12 greased muffin papers (in a pan).

3. Bake at 375 degrees for 29 minutes.

4. Cool for 4 minutes before serving.

Freezing Instructions

5. After cooling, place in zip-lock freezer bag. For the best flavor, heat in microwave or toaster oven before eating.

Nutritional Value: Calories: 200, Total Fat: 39g, Protein: 16g, Total Carbs: 2g, Dietary Fiber: 0g, Sugar: 0, Sodium: 370mg

Black and Blue Smoothie

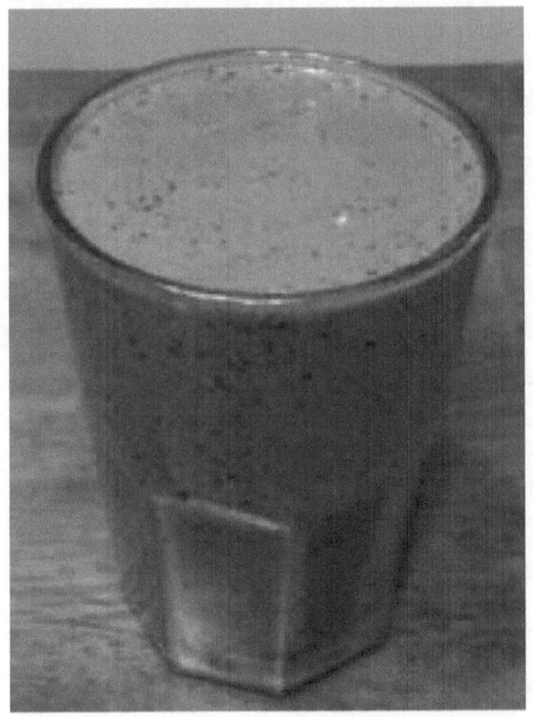

Prep time: 4 minutes

Cook time: 0 minutes

Serves: 1

Ingredients

- ¼ cup Frozen Blueberries

- ¼ cup Frozen Blackberries

- 1 cup unsweetened soy or almond milk

- 1 tablespoon vanilla

- 1 scoop (your choice) vanilla whey protein powder

- 2 packets sweetener of your choice

- 3 tablespoon flaxseeds

Directions

1. Mix the ingredients and emulsify by blending.

2. Pulse four times or until desired thickness.

3. Pour into a glass and enjoy.

4. Combine berries in freezer bags and place in the freezer. Combine sweetener of your choice, flaxseeds, and protein powder in zip-lock bags. Combine milk and vanilla in 1 cup containers in the fridge.

Nutritional Value: Calories: 221, Total Fat: 9.8g, Protein: 21.8g, Total Carbs: 10g, Dietary Fiber: 5.8g, Sugar: 1g, Sodium: 0mg

Breakfast Mexican Omelet

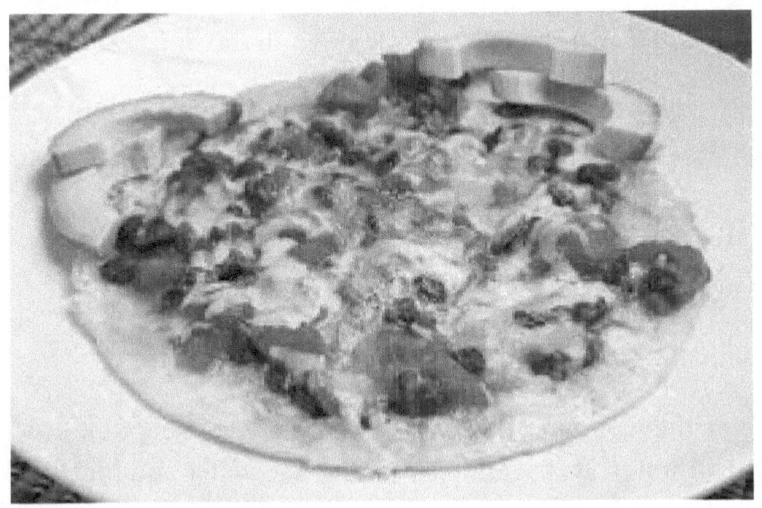

Prep time: 4 minutes

Cook time: 9 minutes

Serves: 1

Ingredients

- ½ tablespoon lime juice

- 2 eggs 1 tablespoon water

- 1 tablespoon crumbled bacon

- 1/2 tablespoon butter

- ¼ avocado

- ½ cup hand-shredded Mexican cheese

- 2 tablespoon Pace Thick and Chunky Medium Salsa

Directions

1. Melt the butter in a microwaveable bowl in the microwave.

2. Quickly whip the wet ingredients in a microwaveable bowl, can be the same bowl as before.

3. Microwave for one minute.

4. Place on warm plate.

5. Top with all the rest of the ingredients.

6. Combine the wet ingredients in a zip-lock bag, except the butter and water. Refrigerate. Combine the water and butter in a zip-lock bag.

Nutritional Value: Calories: 275, Total Fat: 21, Protein: 17g, Total Carbs: 3.2g, Dietary Fiber: 2g, Sugar: 2g, Sodium: 230mg

Cheese Blintz with Blueberries

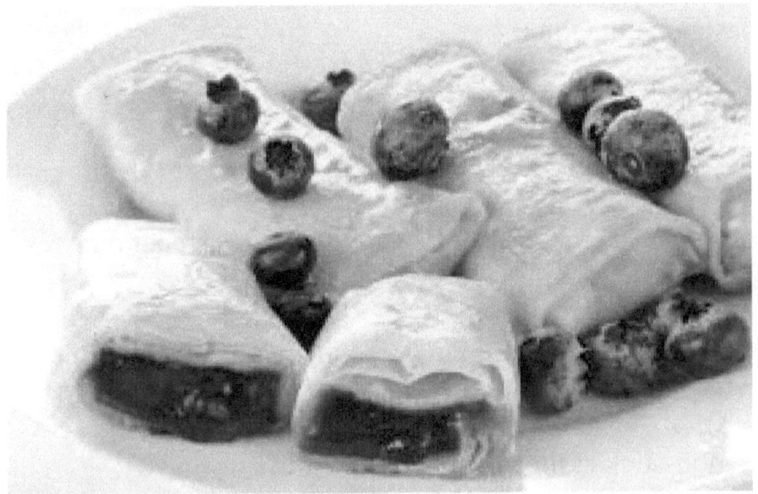

Prep time: 9 minutes

Cook time: 4 minutes

Serves: 1

Ingredients

- 1 medium egg

- 1 tablespoon half & half

- 1 scoop protein shake powder, vanilla

- 1 pat of butter

- 1 tablespoon of olive oil

- 2 tablespoon ricotta cheese

- 1 tablespoon Greek yogurt, plain

- 1 packet sweetener

- 1 tablespoon cinnamon

- ½ cup blueberries

Directions

1. Combine the ricotta cheese, Greek yogurt, sweetener and cinnamon in a bowl, mix well.

2. Combine the egg, protein powder, and cream. Whisk until all lumps are dissolved, and the mixture is well-blended.

3. Coat a non-stick skillet with the olive oil.

4. At medium heat, melt butter in the skillet and pour the batter on top.

5. Swirl the skillet until the batter is evenly distributed. When the batter has set, gently turn the blintz to the other side.

6. Let cook for one minute until the batter is set, but not browned.

7. Gently fold half the blueberries into the filling.

8. Place the filling in the middle of the blitz.

9. Roll into a pancake and serve with the remaining blueberries.

10. Mix the filling and place in the fridge in a covered container. Place the blueberries in a zip-lock bag and place in the freezer.

Nutritional Value: Calories: 427 Total Fat: 23g, Protein: 39g, Total Carbs: 14g, Dietary Fiber: 3g, Sugar: 10g, Sodium: 330mg

Huevos Rancheros

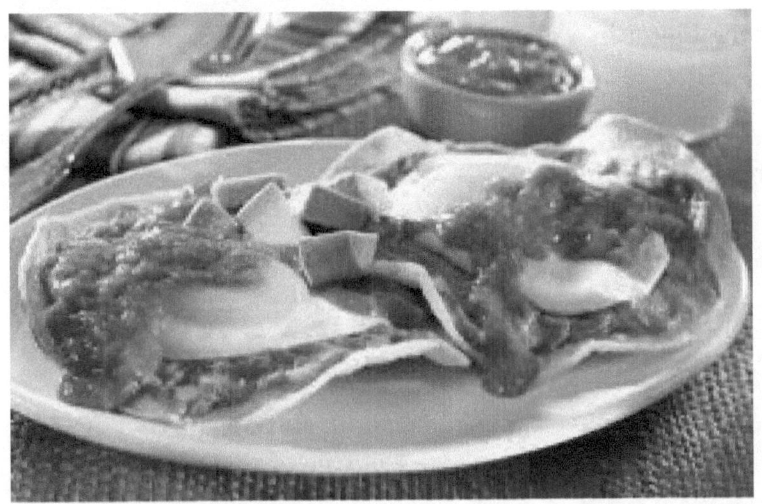

Prep time: 9 minutes

Cook time: 19 minutes

Serves: 4

Ingredients

- 4 oz. cooked ground sirloin

- ½ cup Pace Salsa Verde

- 4 eggs

- 4 slices Canadian bacon

- 4 Tortilla Factory Low Carb Whole Wheat tortillas

- 4 tablespoon water

- 4 tablespoon butter

Directions

1. Melt the butter in a glass bowl.

2. Quickly whip the egg and water with the butter.

3. Microwave 1 minute.

4. Place the tortilla in the microwave for 10 seconds.

5. Layer as follows: Tortilla, Canadian bacon, ground beef, egg, salsa.

6. Place Canadian bacon, cooked sirloin, and salsa into a zip-lock bag. Freeze or refrigerate. Place the tortillas in the fridge to keep them fresh. Add the eggs, etc. when microwaving

Nutritional Value: Calories: 277, Total Fat: 17g, Protein: 20g, Total Carbs: 8g, Dietary Fiber: 13g, Sugar: 3g, Sodium: 720mg

Butter Pecan Waffles

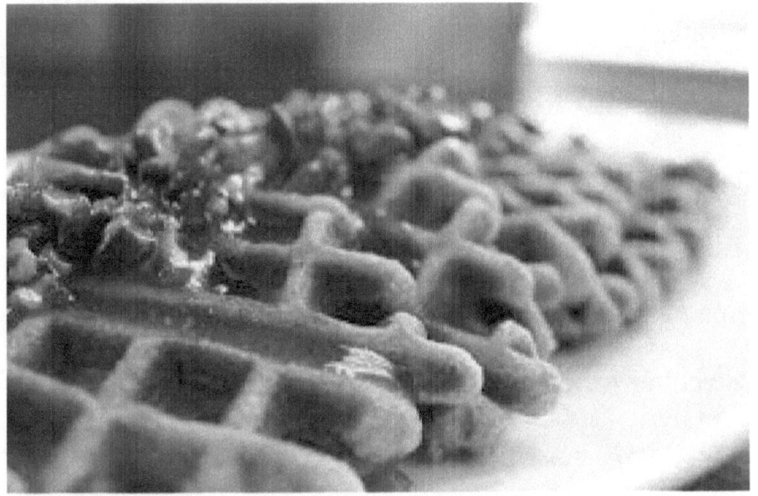

Prep time: 9 minutes

Cook time: 4 minutes

Serves: 8

Ingredients

- 1 cup soy flour

- 2 packets Splenda

- 3 tablespoon baking powder

- ¾ cup buttermilk

- 1 tablespoon butter

- ½ tablespoon baking soda

- 3 eggs

- 2 tablespoon vanilla

- ½ cup water

- 2 tablespoon sugar free butter rum flavoring

- ½ cup pecans

Directions

1. Combine everything except the pecans.

2. Use ¼ c batter for cooking the waffle.

3. Cook until crisp.

4. Top with pecans and sugar free syrup.

5. After the waffle is cool, place 1 per zip-lock bag. Warm by toasting in the toaster.

Nutritional Value: Calories: 181, Total Fat: 13g, Protein: 9g, Total Carbs: 5g, Dietary Fiber: 2g, Sugar: 3g, Sodium: 178mg

Breakfast Casserole

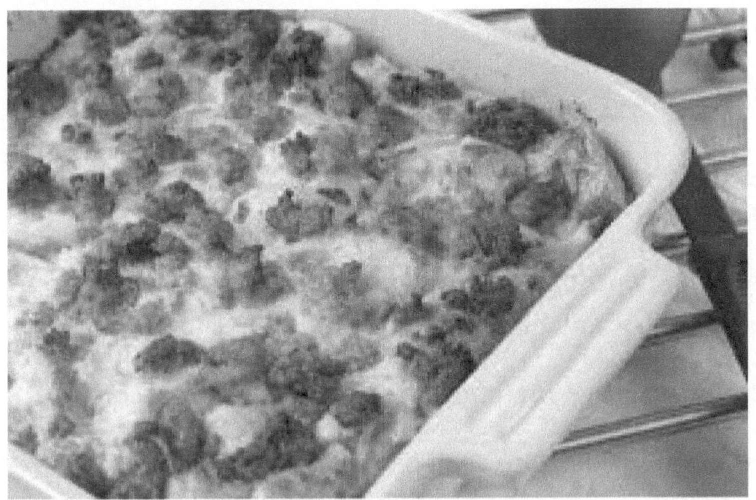

Prep time: 4 minutes

Cook time: 19 minutes

Serves: 4

Ingredients

- 8 oz Sausage, Cooked and Crumbled

- 1 cup hot salsa

- 4 eggs

- 2 chopped green onions

- ¼ cup hand-shredded pepper jack or cheddar cheese

- ½ bell pepper, chopped, your choice of color

Directions

1. Place oven rack to the middle shelf setting.

2. Heat oven to 400 degrees.

3. Cook the peppers until soft.

4. Spray or grease the baking dishes excessively. Eggs stick when baked.

5. Layer ingredients in 4 individual baking dishes, like Corning ware "grab-its," any bakeware that holds one cup servings.

6. Layer with sausage first, then peppers, then cheese.

7. Add one whipped egg to each baking dish. Sprinkle with green onions.

8. Bake for 18 minutes, until eggs are set.

9. Place cooled casseroles in individual freezer bags. Reheat in microwave for 2-3 minutes until hot.

Nutritional Value: Calories: 195, Total Fat: 11g, Protein: 19g, Total Carbs: 3g, Dietary Fiber: 1g, Sugar: 0, Sodium: 112mg

Cinnamon Chocolate Smoothie

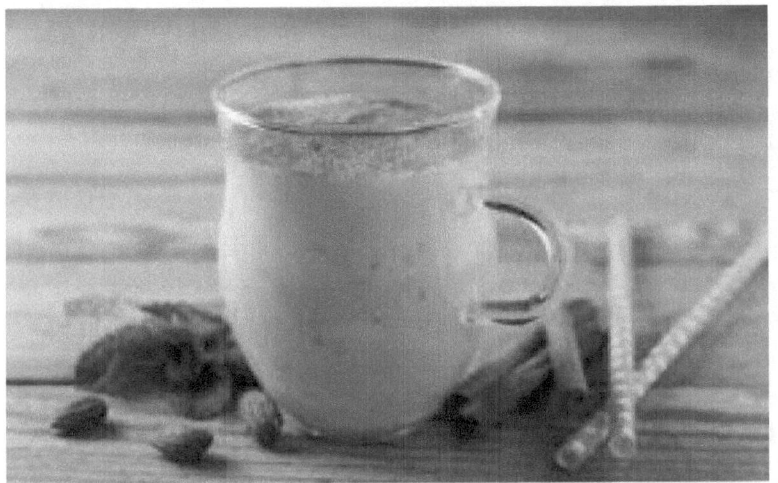

Prep time: 4 minutes

Cook time: 0 minutes

Serves: 1

Ingredients

- ½ cup firm Tofu

- 2 tablespoon cocoa powder

- 1 scoop chocolate protein powder

- 2 tablespoon cinnamon

- 2 sweetener packets

- 1 cup almond milk, unsweetened

- 4 ice cubes

Directions

1. Place all the ingredients in a blender, pulse until desired consistency, and serve.

2. Refrigerate the tofu. Place all the dry ingredients into one snack sized zip-lock bag.

Nutritional Value: Calories: 273, Total Fat: 15g, Protein: 33g, Total Carbs: 9g, Dietary Fiber: 20g, Sugar: 2g, Sodium: 214mg

Chocolate Muffin

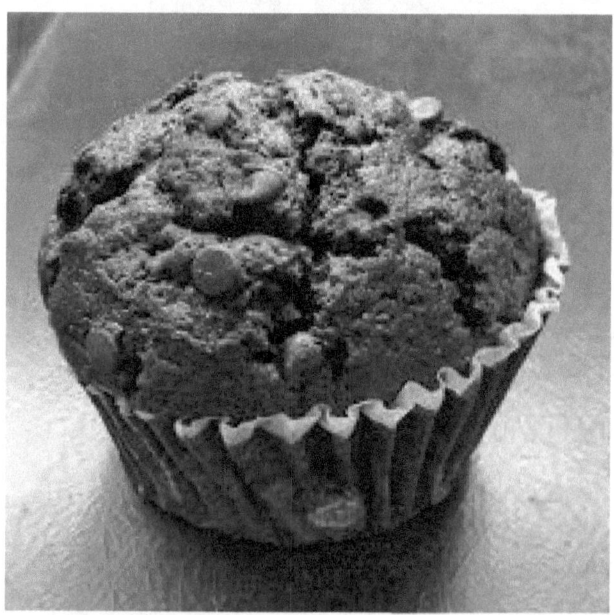

Prep time: 4 minutes

Cook time: 1 minutes

Serves: 1

Ingredients

- 1 tablespoon plain flour

- 1 scoop of Chocolate Protein Powder

- ½ tablespoon baking powder

- 1 tablespoon of cocoa powder

- 2 packets Splenda

- 1 tablespoon butter

- 1 egg

Directions

1. Mix the dry ingredients in a cup

2. Combine the wet ingredients

3. Add the wet ingredients into the cup of dry

4. Microwave for one minute

5. Place individual muffins in a zip-lock bag and place in the freezer. Microwave one minute to thaw and serve.

Nutritional Value: Calories: 207, Total Fat: 24g, Protein: 10g, Total Carbs: 16, Dietary Fiber: 11g, Sugar: 0, Sodium: 308mg

Denver Omelet

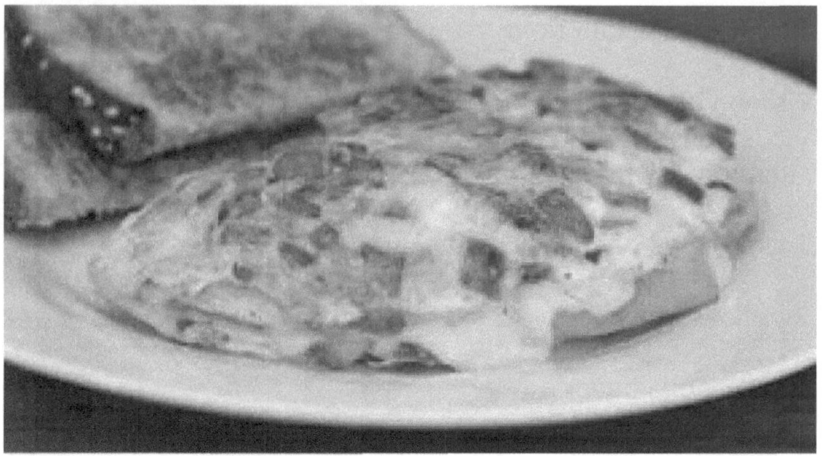

Prep time: 4 minutes

Cook time: 1 minutes

Serves: 1

Ingredients

- 2 tablespoon butter

- ¼ cup chopped onions

- ¼ cup green bell pepper, diced

- ¼ cup halved grape tomatoes

- 2 eggs

- ¼ cup chopped ham

Directions

1. Sautee the onions and bell pepper, with the butter, in a small skillet.

2. Whip the eggs and mix the ingredients in a bowl.

3. Microwave for one minute.

4. Pre-cook the peppers and onions and place in zip-lock freezer bags by portions, add the ham to the bags. Freeze. The night before making, place the peppers mix in the fridge to thaw or microwave for one minute before adding to the whipped egg to make.

Nutritional Value: Calories: 605, Total Fat: 46g, Protein: 39g, Total Carbs: 6g, Dietary Fiber: 2g, Sugar: 0g, Sodium: 380mg

Almond Joy Microwave Muffin

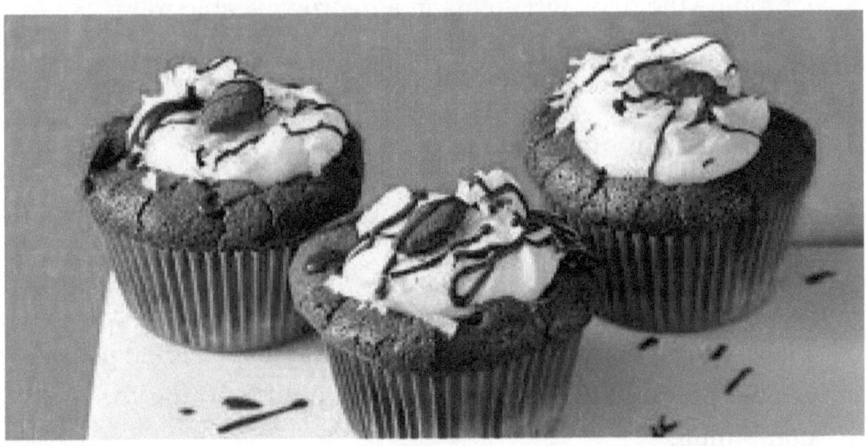

Prep time: 3 minutes

Cook time: 1 minutes

Serves: 1

Ingredients

- 2 tablespoon almond flour

- 1 tablespoon Coconut Flour

- 1 packet Splenda

- 1/4 tablespoon Baking Powder

- Sprinkle with Salt

- 1 Egg

- 1 tablespoon butter

- 1 tablespoon cocoa

Directions

1. Combine the dry ingredients in a microwaveable mug.

2. Quickly whip the egg and the oil together.

3. Stir into the dry mixture.

4. Microwave on high for 1 minute.

5. Toast with butter.

6. Place all dry ingredients in zip-lock baggies, 1 recipe per bag. Do not premix the eggs and oil. Wait until morning for combining.

Nutritional Value: Calories: 207, Total Fat: 16.8g, Protein: 9.7g, Total Carbs: 3.7g, Dietary Fiber: 3, Sugar: 0, Sodium: 300mg

Ham Rollups

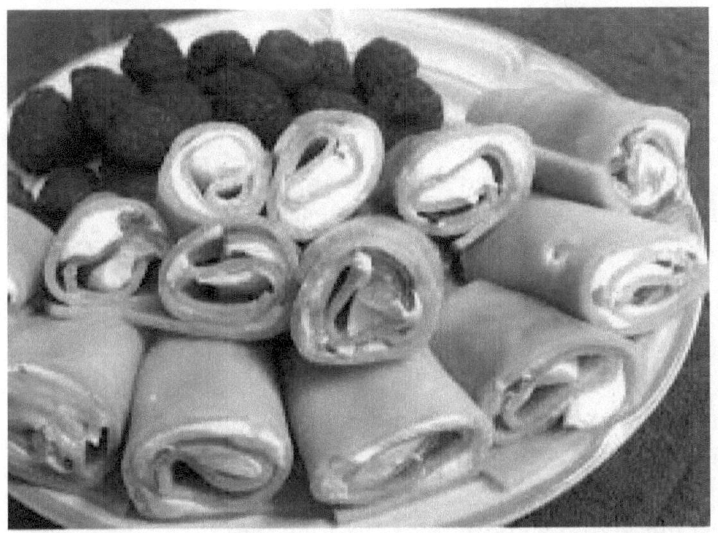

Prep time: 9 minutes

Cook time: 0 minutes

Serves: 6

Ingredients

- 6 Tortilla Factory low carb whole wheat tortillas

- 8 oz. whipped cream cheese

- 6 slices ham, the rectangular kind, cut in half

- ½ cup pickle dill relish

- 2 tablespoon mayonnaise

- 2 tablespoon Dijon mustard

Directions

1. Combine cream cheese, dill relish, mustard and mayo in a bowl.

2. Lay one tortilla out on waxed paper or saran wrap.

3. Place one slice of ham on top.

4. Spread ham slices with the cream cheese mixture.

5. Roll the entire piece up.

6. Cut in half.

7. Refrigerate until serving, 1 whole tortilla is one serving, so if cut in half, is still one serving.

8. Place serving size per individual zip-lock bag.

Nutritional Value: Calories: 228, Total Fat: 18g, Protein: 18g, Total Carbs: 6g, Dietary Fiber: 7g, Sugar: 0g, Sodium: 358mg

Junior Mint Shake

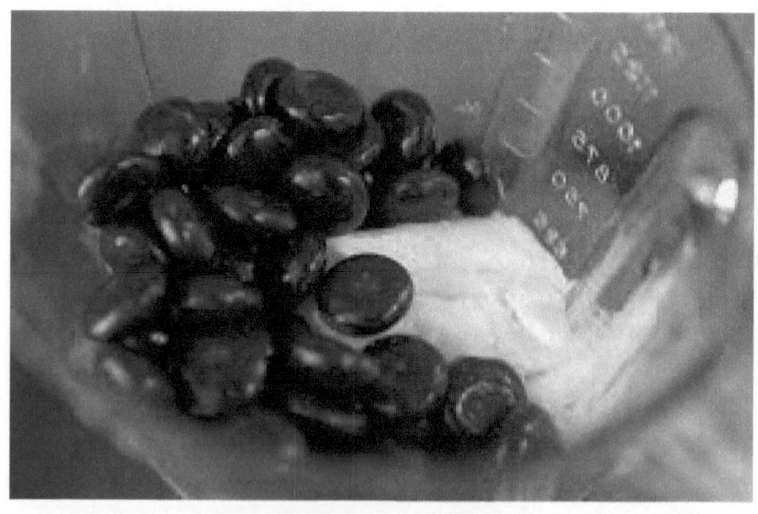

Prep time: 4 minutes

Cook time: 0

Serves: 1

Ingredients

- 2 tablespoon cocoa

- 6 oz. COLD water

- ¼ cup protein powder or chocolate

- 3 drops peppermint flavoring

- ½ cup cottage cheese

- 2 packets sweetener

- 5 ice cubes

Directions

1. Mix the ingredients and emulsify by blending.

2. Blend until thick.

3. Combine dry ingredients and place in zip-lock bag. Combine cottage cheese and sweetener and refrigerate.

Nutritional Value: Calories: 200, Total Fat: 2g, Protein: 39g, Total Carbs: 7g, Dietary Fiber: 1g, Sugar: 3g, Sodium: 348mg

Spicy Deviled Eggs

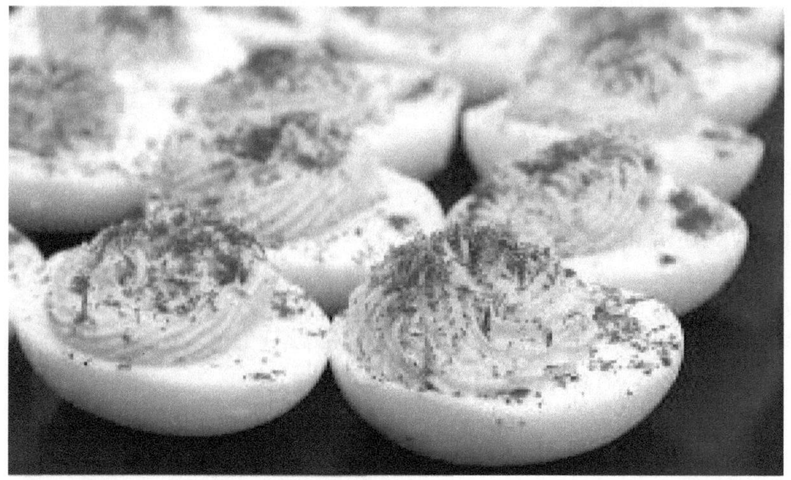

Prep time: 9 minutes

Cook time: 11 minutes

Serves: 2

Ingredients

- 4 hard-boiled eggs

- 2 tablespoon mayonnaise

- 1 tablespoon spicy brown mustard

- 1 tablespoon diced green chilies

Directions

1. Boil the eggs for 9 minutes.

2. Slice the eggs in half.

3. Scoop out the yolks.

4. Mix the yolks, the mayo, the mustard and the chilies.

5. Place back in the center of the egg whites.

6. Boil the eggs in advance and place in the fridge.

Nutritional Value: Calories: 202, Total Fat: 15g, Protein: 12g, Total Carbs: 3, Dietary Fiber: 0g, Sugar: 2g, Sodium: 20mg

Chapter 10: Lunch

Italian Eggplant Lasagna

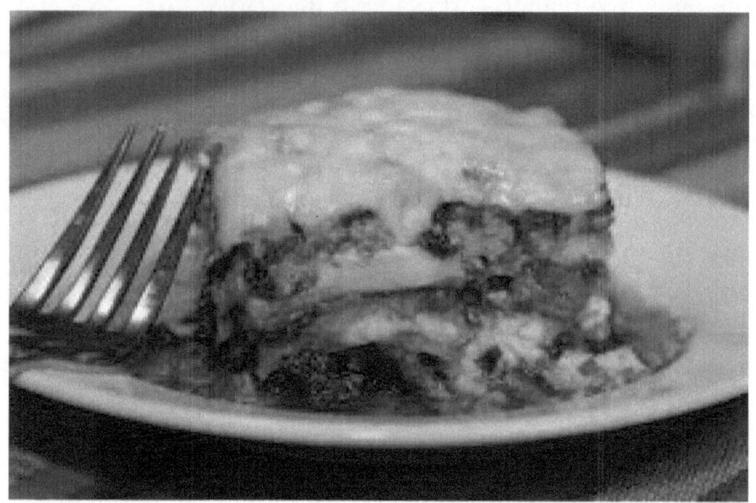

Prep time: 1 Hour and 45 Minutes

Serves: 8

Ingredients:

- 1 eggplant, sliced thinly

- 2 tablespoons of salt

- 6 tablespoon of extra virgin olive oil

- 1 pound of Italian sausage

- 2 cups of ricotta cheese

- 2 cups of marinara sauce

- 3 cups of mozzarella cheese, shredded

- 2 cups of Parmesan cheese, grated

Directions:

1. Place the eggplant slices on a flat surface. Season with a dash of salt and set aside to sit for 20 to 30 minutes.

2. Preheat the oven to 400 degrees.

3. Pat dry the paper towels with a sheet of paper towels.

4. Drizzle the olive oil over the eggplant slices and place onto a large baking sheet. Place into the oven to roast for 10 minutes.

5. While the eggplant slices are roasting place a large skillet over medium heat. Add in the Italian sausage and cook for 10 to 12 minutes or until cooked through. Remove and set aside.

6. Reduce the temperature in the oven to 375 degrees.

7. Then use a large bowl and add in the Italian sausage and ricotta cheese. Stir well to mix. Pour half a cup of this mixture into the bottom of a large greased baking dish. Lay down 1/3 of the eggplant slices into the baking dish. Repeat the layers. Top off with the marinara sauce, mozzarella cheese and Parmesan cheese.

8. Cover the baking dish with a sheet of aluminum foil. Place into the oven to bake for 30 to 40 minutes. Remove the aluminum foil and continue to bake for another 10 minutes or until browned.

9. Remove from the oven and allow cooling for 20 minutes before serving.

Nutritional Value: Calories: 667, Fat: 51 grams, Carbs: 14 grams, Protein: 38 grams

Chicken Piccata

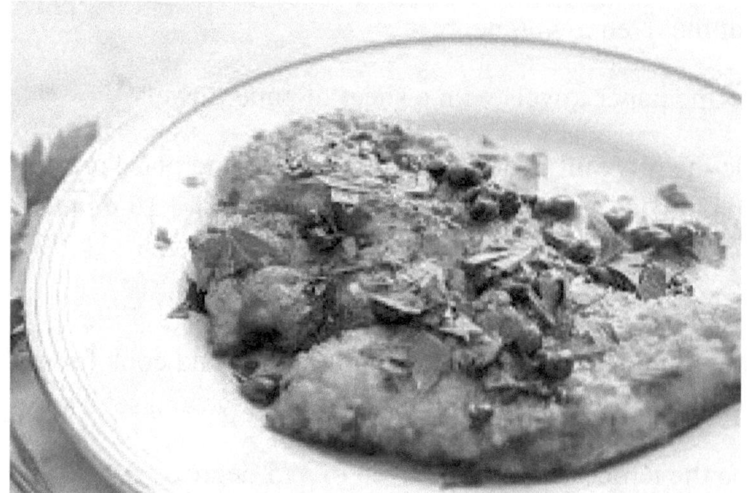

Prep time: 20 Minutes

Serves: 4

Ingredients:

- 4 chicken thighs, a dash of salt and black pepper

- 4 tablespoon of extra virgin olive oil

- 6 ounces of butter, soft

- ¼ cup of white wine, dried

- ¼ cup of lemon juice, fresh

- ½ cup of chicken stock

- ¼ cup of capers, brined

- 4 tablespoons of heavy cream

- ¼ cup of parsley, fresh and chopped

Directions:

1. Season the chicken thighs with a dash of salt and black pepper.

2. Place a large saucepan over medium to high heat. Add in the extra virgin olive oil and two tablespoons of soft butter. Once the butter begins to simmer add in the chicken thighs. Cook for 5 minutes on each side or until cooked through. Remove from the saucepan and transfer to a large plate.

3. Add the dried white wine into the saucepan and deglaze the pan.

4. Add in the fresh lemon juice, chicken stock and capers. Stir well to mix and bring the mixture to a boil. Once boiling reduces the heat to low.

5. Add the chicken back into the saucepan. Allow to simmer for 5 minutes.

6. Transfer the chicken back into a large plate.

7. Add the heavy cream and remaining butter into the saucepan. Season with a dash of salt and black pepper. Whisk to mix.

8. Pour the sauce over the chicken. Serve with a garnish of parsley.

Nutritional Value: Calories: 468, Fat: 39 grams, Carbs: 3.6 grams, Protein: 28 grams

Indian Chicken Curry

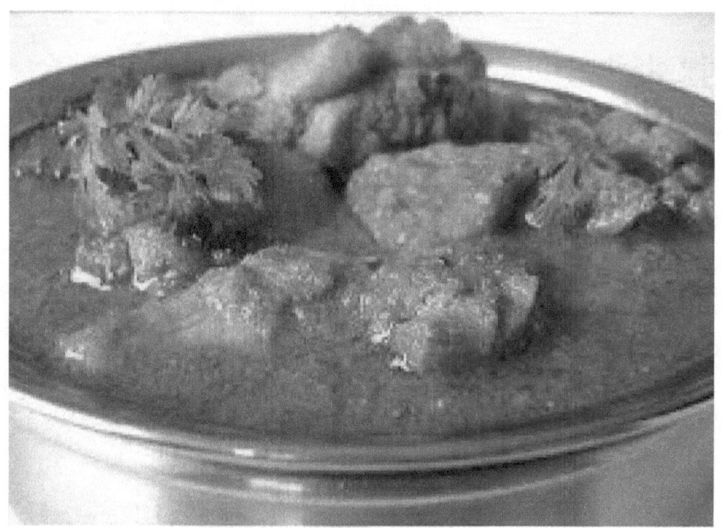

Prep Time: 2 Hours

Serves: 8

Ingredients:

- 6 chicken thighs, cut into small pieces

- 1 onion, diced

- 4 cloves of garlic, minced

- 1 tablespoon of salt

- 2 tablespoon of red curry paste

- 2 tablespoons of curry, powdered

- 2 tablespoon of soy sauce

- 5 drops of Stevia

- 3 tablespoons of cilantro, fresh, chopped and extra for garnish

- ¼ cup of extra virgin olive oil

- 3 tablespoon of coconut oil

- ½ cup of heavy cream

- 2 tablespoons of cornstarch

- 2 tablespoons of cold water

- 1 lime, fresh and juice only

Directions:

1. Use a large bowl and add in the chicken thigh pieces, onion, garlic, dash of salt, red curry paste, powdered curry, soy sauce, stevia, cilantro and extra virgin olive oil. Stir well to mix.

2. Cover the bowl and set into the fridge to marinate for 1 hour.

3. After this time place a large skillet over medium to high heat. Add in the coconut oil and once the oil is hot enough add in the marinated chicken. Cook for 8 to 10 minutes or until the chicken is cooked through.

4. Pour in the coconut milk and bring the mixture to a boil. Once boiling reduce the heat to low. Cover and cook for 30

to 40 minutes. Make sure to stir the chicken every 5 to 10 minutes.

5. Add in the heavy cream after this time and increase the heat to high. Bring the mixture to a boil.

6. While the mixture is coming to a boil add the cornstarch and water into a small bowl. Whisk to make a slurry and pour into the chicken mixture. Stir well to mix and cook for 5 minutes or until thick in consistency.

7. Add in the fresh lime juice and a dash of salt.

8. Remove from heat and serve.

Nutritional Value: Calories: 408, Fat: 32 grams, Carbs: 7 grams, Protein: 23 grams

No Bake Cheesecake

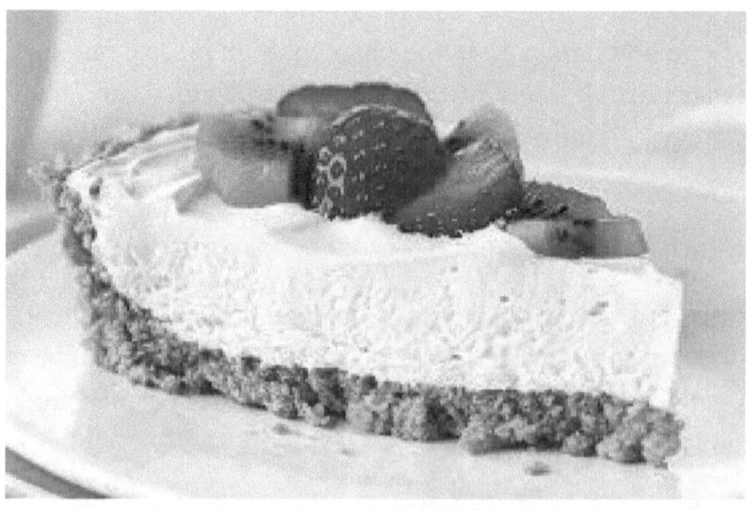

Prep Time: 6 Hours and 15 Minutes

Serves: 12

Ingredients:

- ½ cup of almond flour

- ¼ cup of butter, melted

- 16 ounces of cream cheese, soft

- ¾ cup of artificial sweetener

- ½ tablespoon of pure vanilla

- ½ tablespoon of lemon juice, fresh

- ½ tablespoon of salt

Directions:

1. Spray a muffin pan with cooking spray and line with paper muffin lines.

2. Use a large bowl and add in the almond flour and butter. Stir well until mixed. Pour this mixture into the bottom of each muffin cup. Press flat to make a crust.

3. Use a separate bowl and add in the cream cheese, artificial sweetener, pure vanilla, fresh lemon juice and dash of salt. Beat with an electric mixer until creamy in consistency. Pour this mixture over the crusts.

4. Place the muffin pan into the freezer to freeze for 2 hours.

5. Remove after this time and transfer into the fridge to thaw for 3 to 4 hours. Serve. Flank Steak Stuffed with Pancetta and

Goat Cheese This is a great tasting keto friendly dish you can make for lunch or dinner.

Nutritional Value: Calories: 195, Fat: 19 grams, Carbs: 3 grams, Protein: 3 grams

Chicken Lettuce Wraps

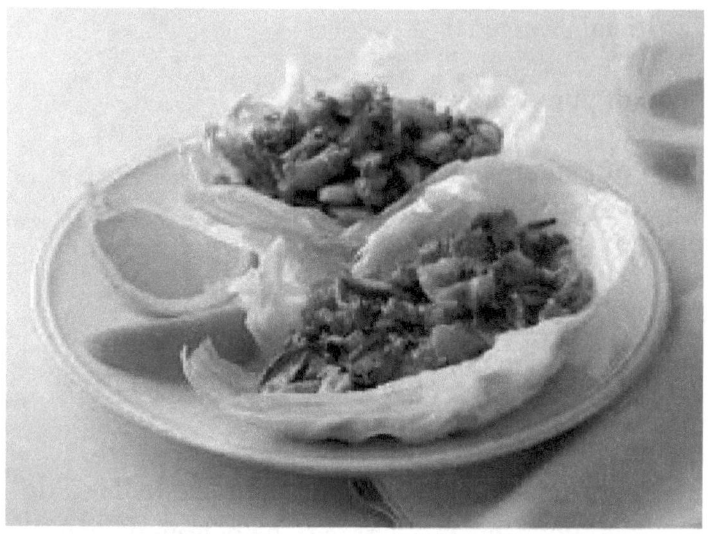

Prep time: 10minutes

Cook time: 10minutes

Serves: 1

Ingredients

- 1 chicken breast, boneless, diced into 1-inch size pieces

- 1 cup diced or sliced fresh mushrooms

- ½ cup diced water chestnuts (from a can, drained)

- 1 tablespoon of olive oil

- 1 tablespoon onion, minced

- 1 tablespoon minced garlic

- 1 tablespoon teriyaki sauce

- garlic powder, only a dash

- onion powder, just a dash

- oregano, one dash

- cayenne pepper, a small dash

- salt /pepper

Directions

1. Mix the ingredients and cook in a skillet until the chicken is done, about 10 minutes.

2. Shred the chicken

3. Place in leaves and roll

4. Place all ingredients into one freezer bag except the lettuce. Microwave one minute and serve.

Nutritional Value: Calories: 145, Total Fat: 1g, Protein: 35g, Dietary Fiber: 1g, Total Carbs: 4g, Sugar: 0g, Sodium: 100mg

Stuffed with goat cheese,

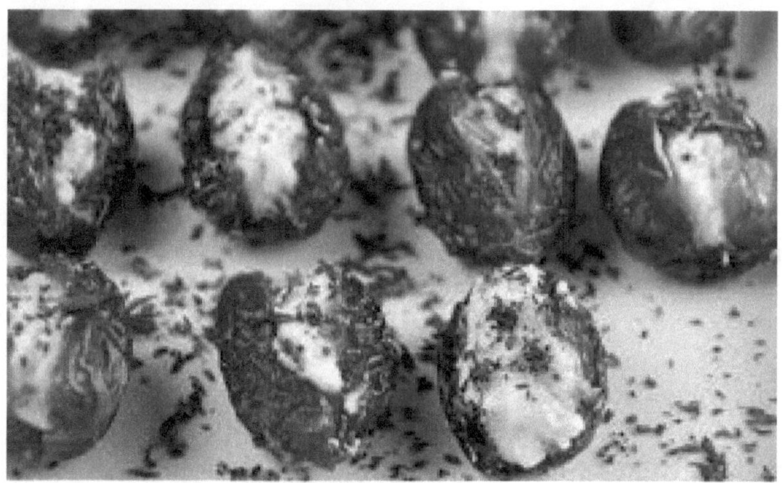

Prep Time: 5 Hours and 30 Minutes

Serves: 4

Ingredients:

- ¼ cup of red wine

- ¼ cup of balsamic vinegar

- 2 tablespoon of Dijon mustard

- 2 tablespoon of soy sauce

- 1 cup of extra virgin olive oil

- 4 cloves of garlic, peeled and thinly sliced

- 1 tablespoon of Salt Dash black pepper

- 1, 2 to 3 pounds of flank steak

Ingredients for the stuffing:

- ½ cup of pancetta, cooked and chopped

- 8 ounces of goat cheese

- 3 cups of spinach, drained and excess liquid drained

Directions:

1. Use a large bowl and add in the red wine, vinegar, mustard, soy sauce, olive oil, garlic and dash of salt and black pepper. Whisk until mixed.

2. Add in the flank steak and cover. Set in the fridge to marinate for 4 hours.

3. Place a large saucepan over low heat. Chop the pancetta and place into the saucepan. Cook for 20 to 30 minutes. Drain the excess fat and set the pancetta aside.

4. Add the spinach into the saucepan and cook for 1 to 2 minutes or until fragrant. Remove from the pan and squeeze out the excess liquid. Add into a bowl with the pancetta and goat cheese. Stir well to mix.

5. Remove the flank steak from the marinade and place onto a flat surface. Beat with a meat mallet until ¼ inch in thickness.

6. Spread the stuffing onto the flank steak. Roll and tie with twine to seal. Season with a dash of salt and black pepper.

7. Heat up the oven to 400 degrees.

8. Place the rolled flank steak onto a large baking sheet and drizzle a few drops of olive oil over the top.

9. Place into the oven to bake for 15 to 25 minutes or until cooked through. Remove and allow to rest for 15 minutes before serving.

Nutritional Value: Calories: 646, Fat: 58 grams, Carbs: 4 grams, Protein: 27 grams

Chili Mac

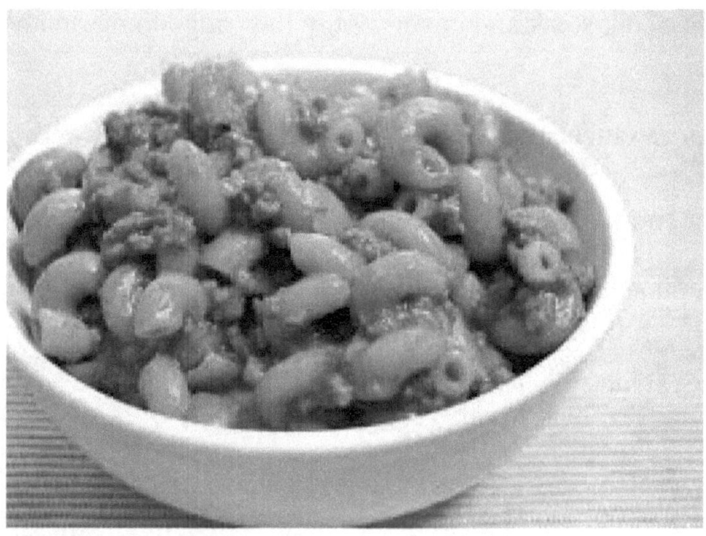

Prep time: 9 minutes

Cook time: 9 minutes

Serves: 4

Ingredients

- 1 lbs. ground Sirloin

- 1 chopped Onion

- 1 Chili Seasoning Mix, packet

- 1 cup tomato sauce

- 1 small can of Chunky Diced Tomatoes & Green Chilies

- 1 cup hand-shredded sharp cheddar

- 1 packet Splenda

- ½ cup Barilla Protein Plus Elbow macaroni

Directions

1. Boil Barilla Protein Plus Elbow macaroni until done, drain.

2. Brown the sirloin and onions in a large skillet.

3. Add the pasta, tomato sauce, diced tomatoes and green chilies, and chili seasoning mix.

4. Taste to see if you need to add water.

5. Serve in 4 bowls, topping each bowl with the cheddar cheese.

6. Place in four containers with lids, freeze. Microwave 2 minutes to thaw.

Nutritional Value: Calories: 480, Total Fat: 24g, Protein: 36g, Total Carbs: g, 25Dietary Fiber: 6g, Sugar: 4g, Sodium: 995mg

Chicken Quesadillas

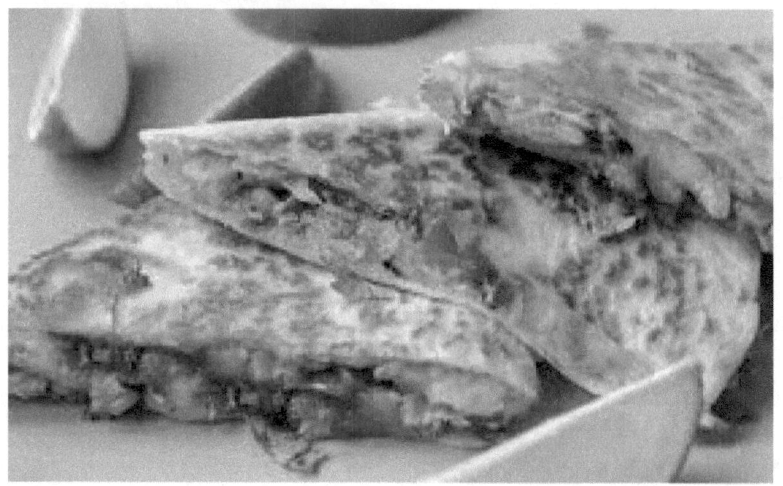

Prep time: 4 minutes

Cook time: 4 minutes

Serves: 4

Ingredients

- 1 cup pepper jack cheese, hand-shredded

- 8 tortillas Tortilla Factory Low Carb Whole Wheat Tortillas

- 8 oz. cooked and shredded Chicken Breast

- 1 chopped and Roasted Bell Pepper

- 2 tablespoon Cilantro

- 2 tablespoon Butter

- 1 cup plain Greek yogurt

Directions

1. Place ½ pat of butter in a skillet

2. Mix all the ingredients in a bowl except the yogurt

3. Place meat ingredients inside tortillas

4. Toast each side

5. Cut into 4 wedges

6. Top with yogurt and salsa, if desired

7. Freeze in zip-lock bags. Place the yogurt in the fridge. Heat one minute in the microwave to thaw.

Nutritional Value: Calories: 425g, Total Fat: 25g, Protein: 44g, Total Carbs: 10g, Dietary Fiber: 9g, Sugar: 2g, Sodium: 186mg

Cobb Salad

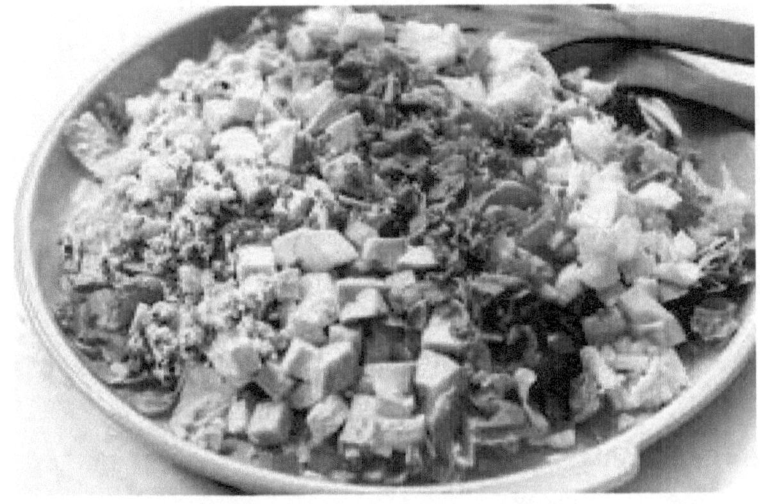

Prep time: 9 minutes

Cook time: 9 minutes

Serves: 1

Ingredients

- 1 slice of Bacon or 1 tablespoon real bacon bits

- 1 grilled Chicken Breast, which has been cut into thin strips

- 1 cup Spring Mix Salad

- 1/2 cup grape tomatoes, sliced in half

- ½ avocado, sliced into small moons

- ¼ cup pepper jack cheese, hand-shredded

- 2 tablespoon Ken's Buttermilk Ranch Dressing

Directions

1. Assemble ingredients by sections.

2. Cover the entire bottom of the plate with lettuce.

3. In one corner (relative if you have a round plate) place the tomatoes.

4. In the opposite section place the avocado strips in a fan shape.

5. In the third section place the bacon bits.

6. In the fourth section place the hand-shredded cheese. In the center place the chicken.

7. Drizzle with the salad dressing and serve.

8. The chicken can be frozen in a zip-lock bag. Microwave 1 minute to serve. The salad can be combined in one bowl or packed in individual containers and placed in the fridge.

Nutritional Value: Calories: 561, Total Fat: 34g, Protein: 51g, Total Carbs: 3.9g, Dietary Fiber: 6g, Sugar: 1g, Sodium: 802mg

Seven Layer Salad

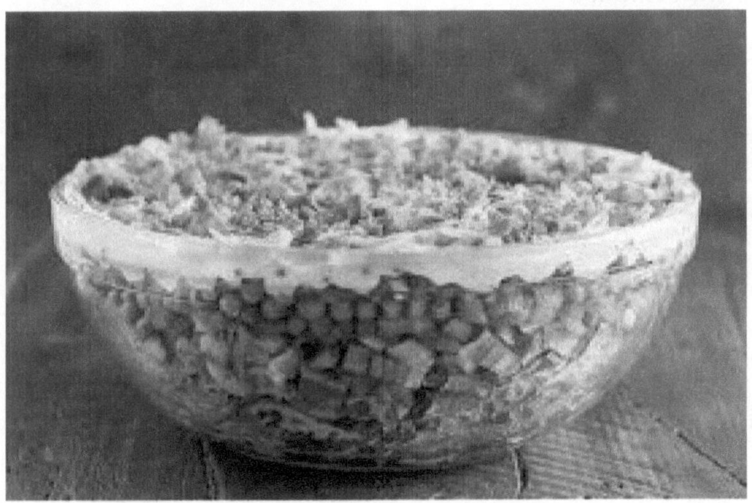

Prep time: 14 minutes

Cook time: 9 minutes

Serves: 10

Ingredients

- 4 cups shredded butter lettuce

- 4 cups shredded romaine lettuce

- 1 cup peas

- 1 cup diced bell peppers, red and yellow

- 1 cup grape tomatoes, halved

- 1 cup sliced celery

- ½ cup red onion

- ¾ cup Greek yogurt

- ¾ cup mayonnaise

- 3 hard-boiled eggs

- 2 teaspoons cider vinegar

- 1 packet Splenda

- ¼ teaspoon garlic salt

- ½ cup pepper-jack cheese, hand-shredded

- 3 strips cooked bacon, crumbled

Directions

1. Using a large glass pan, 9x13 sized, layer the two lettuces.

2. Layer the peas, then the peppers, then the tomatoes, celery and onion.

3. Place the diced eggs next.

4. Combine the dressing ingredients: yogurt, mayonnaise, vinegar, garlic salt, Splenda, and a dash of black pepper.

5. Spread the dressing over the salad.

6. Garnish with the pepper-jack cheese and bacon.

7. Place in one cup containers. Close with a lid and refrigerate.

Nutritional Value: Calories: 136, Total Fat: 7g, Protein: 2g, Total Carbs: 9g, Dietary Fiber: 2g, Sugar: 0g, Sodium: 324mg

Shrimp and Cucumber Salad

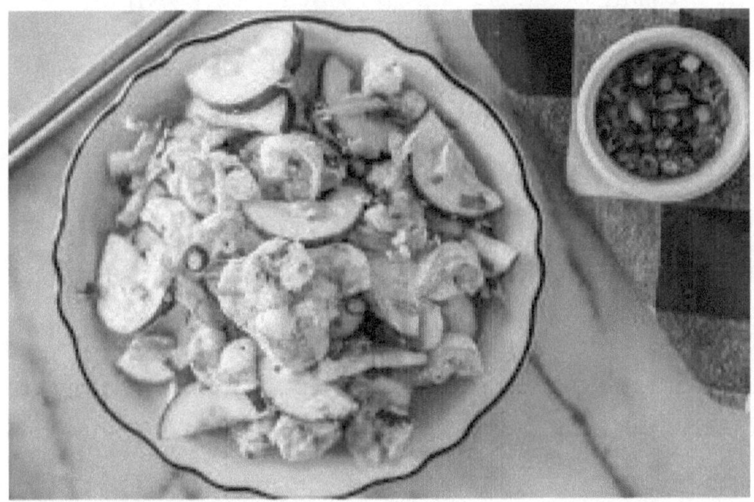

Prep time: 4 minutes

Cook time: 0 minutes

Serves: 4

Ingredients

- 2 English cucumbers

- 1/4 cup of red wine vinegar

- 2 tablespoons of Splenda

- 1/4 tablespoon salt

- ½ cup cooked shrimp

Directions

1. Peel the cucumbers so that they have stripes down the side.

2. Slice the cucumbers as thin as you can.

3. Mix the dressing of sugar, salt, and vinegar very well

4. Place the cucumbers on a plate

5. Place the shrimp on top

6. Add the dressing and serve.

7. Create the entire salad and place in a covered container in the fridge. Will keep 2 days.

Nutritional Value: Calories: 26g, Total Fat: 0g, Protein: 2g, Total Carbs: 3g, Dietary Fiber: 2g, Sugar: 2g, Sodium: 157mg

Feta Cucumber Salad

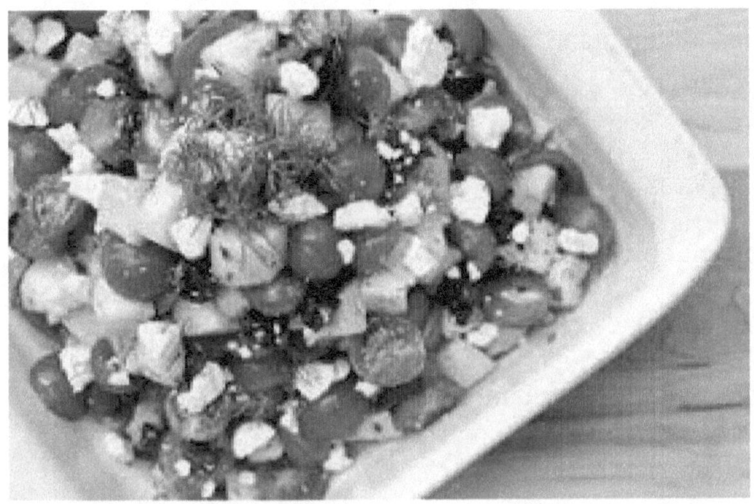

Prep time: 14 minutes

Cook time: none

Serves: 4

Ingredients

- 1 head of leaf lettuce, coarsely chopped

- 1 cup baby spinach, trimmed, coarsely chopped

- ½ cup diced red onion

- 1 cup of grape tomatoes, sliced in half

- ¼ cup Feta cheese, crumbled

- 2 cups plain Greek Yogurt

- 2 tablespoons of garlic powder

- 1 tablespoon dill

- 2 tablespoon lemon juice

- 2 English cucumbers, chopped with peels on

- 2 tablespoon olive oil

- ¼ tablespoon black pepper

- 1 small can black olives, sliced and drained (2.25 oz. can)

- ½ tablespoon mint or 3 mint leaves

Directions

1. Combine Greek yogurt, dill, garlic powder, mint, lemon juice, olive oil, ½ cup diced cucumber, and black pepper and emulsify by blending.

2. Taste and add salt. Add water by tablespoons if too thick.

3. Arrange on 4 plates the lettuce and spinach, tomatoes, cucumbers, and black olives.

4. Pour the dressing over the salad.

5. Top with the feta cheese.

6. Mix the salad dressing and place in fridge in closed containers. Mix the salad and bag or place in covered containers in the fridge.

7. Place the feta cheese in a zip-lock bag in the fridge.

Nutritional Value: Calories: 142, Total Fat: 10g, Protein: 4g, Total Carbs: 7g, Dietary Fiber: 3g, Sugar: 0g, Sodium: 144mg

Chapter 11: Dinner

Chicken Chow Mein Stir Fry

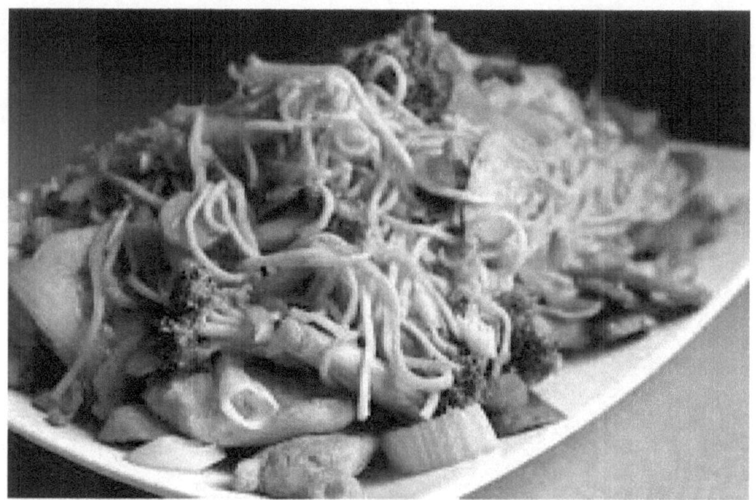

Prep time: 9 minutes

Cook time: 14 minutes

Serves: 4

Ingredients

- 1/2 cup sliced onion

- 2 tablespoons of Oil, sesame garlic flavored

- 4 cups shredded Bok-Choy

- 1 cup Sugar Snap Peas

- 1 cup fresh bean sprouts

- 3 stalks Celery, chopped

- 1 1/2 tablespoon minced Garlic

- 1 packet Splenda

- 1 cup Broth, chicken

- 2 tablespoon Soy Sauce

- 1 tablespoon ginger, freshly minced

- 1 tablespoon cornstarch

- 4 boneless Chicken Breasts, cooked/sliced thinly

Directions

1. Place the Bok-Choy, peas, celery in a skillet with 1 T garlic oil.

2. Stir fry until Bok-Choy is softened to liking.

3. Add remaining ingredients except for the cornstarch.

4. If too thin, stir cornstarch into ½ cup cold water. When smooth pour into skillet.

5. Bring cornstarch and Chow Mein to a one-minute boil. Turn off the heat source.

6. Stir sauce then for wait 4 minutes to serve, after the Chow Mein has thickened.

7. Freeze in covered containers. Heat for 2 minutes in the microwave before serving.

Nutritional Value: Calories: 368, Total Fat: 18g, Protein: 42g, Total Carbs: 12g, Dietary Fiber: 16g, Sugar: 6g, Sodium: 746mg

Chicken Relleno Casserole

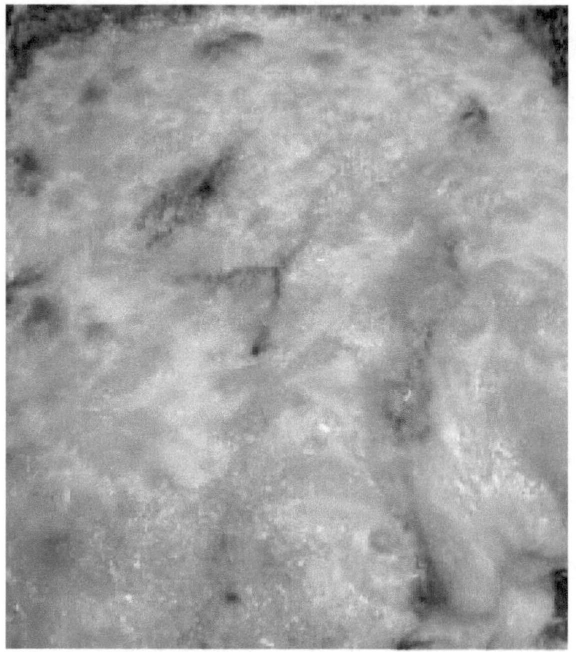

Prep time: 19 minutes

Cook time: 29 minutes

Serves: 6

Ingredients

- 6 Tortilla Factory low-carb whole wheat tortillas, torn into small pieces

- 1 ½ cups hand-shredded cheese, Mexican

- 1 beaten egg

- 1 cup milk

- 2 cups cooked chicken, shredded

- 1 can of Ro-Tel

- ½ cup Salsa Verde

Directions

1. Grease an 8 x 8 glass baking dish

2. Heat oven to 375 degrees

3. Combine everything together, but reserve ½ cup of the cheese

4. Bake it for 29 minutes

5. Take it out of oven and add ½ cup cheese

6. Broil for about 2 minutes to melt the cheese

7. Let the casserole cool. Slice into 6 pieces and place in freezer containers, (1 cup with a lid) Freeze. Microwave for 2 minutes to serve. Top with sour cream, if desired.

Nutritional Value: Calories: 265, Total Fat: 16g, Protein: 20g, Total Carbs: 18g, Dietary Fiber: 10g, Sugar: 0g, Sodium: 708mg

Kabobs with Peanut Curry Sauce

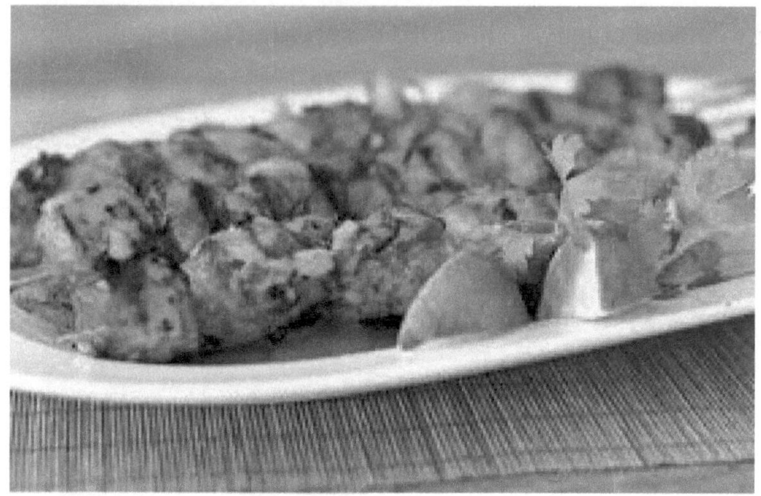

Prep time: 9 minutes

Cook time: 9 minutes

Serves: 4

Ingredients

- 1 cup Cream

- 4 tablespoons of Curry Powder

- 1 1/2 tablespoon Cumin

- 1 1/2 tablespoon Salt

- 1 T minced garlic

- 1/3 cup Peanut Butter, sugar-free

- 2 tablespoon Lime Juice

- 3 tablespoon Water

- 1/2 small Onion, diced

- 2 tablespoon Soy Sauce

- 1 packet Splenda

- 8 oz. boneless, cooked Chicken Breast

- 8 oz. pork tenderloin

Directions

1. Blend together cream, onion, 2 tablespoon garlic, curry and cumin powder, and salt.

2. Slice the meats into 1inch pieces.

3. Place the cream sauce into a bowl and put in the chicken and tenderloin to marinate. Let rest in sauce for 14 minutes.

4. Blend peanut butter, water, 1 tablespoon garlic, lime juice, soy sauce, and Splenda. This is your peanut dipping sauce. Remove the meats and thread on skewers. Broil or grill 4 minutes per side until meat is done.

5. Serve with dipping sauce.

6. Place the meat into zip-lock bags and freeze.

7. Place the peanut sauce and the cream sauce in the fridge in covered containers.

Pizza

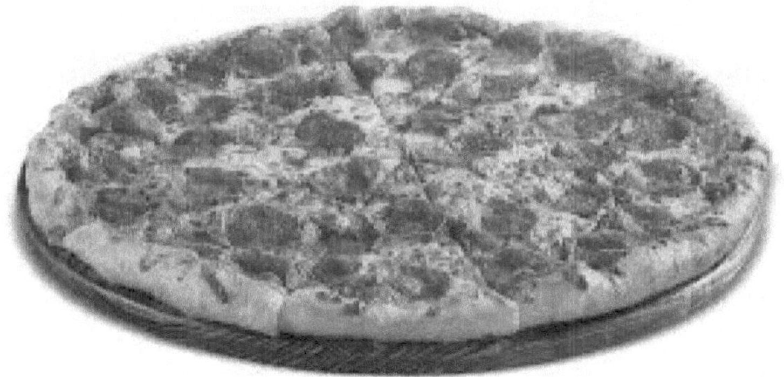

Prep time: 4 minutes

Cook time: 4 minutes

Serves: 1

Ingredients

- 1 Tortilla Factory low carb whole wheat tortilla

- ¼ cup mozzarella cheese, hand-shredded

- ¼ cup tomato paste

- a sprinkle of Italian seasoning

- sprinkle with garlic salt

- Cut the broccoli, spinach, mushrooms, peppers, and onions you like for toppings

Directions

1. Turn broiler on in oven or toaster oven

2. Spread tortilla with tomato paste

3. Sprinkle seasoning on the paste

4. Add the cheese

5. Add the veggies

6. Broil or toast 1-4 minutes until crust is crunchy and cheese melted

7. Place when cooled into individual freezer bags. Microwave for 1 minute to refresh.

Nutritional Value: Calories: 155, Total Fat: 7g, Protein: 13g, Total Carbs: 18g, Dietary Fiber: 10g, Sugar: 2g, Sodium: 741mg

Sriracha Tuna Kabobs

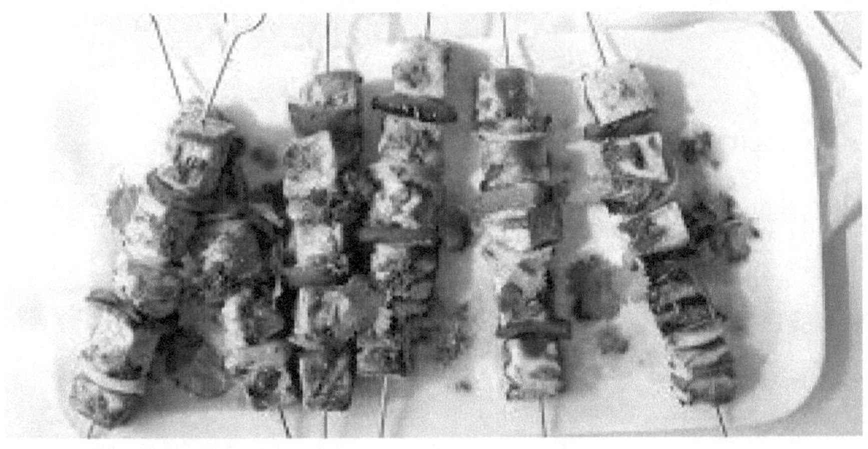

Prep time: 4 minutes

Cook time: 9 minutes

Serves: 4

Ingredients

- 4 tablespoon Huy Fong chili garlic sauce

- 1 tablespoon sesame oil infused with garlic

- 1 tablespoon ginger, fresh, grated

- 1 tablespoon garlic, minced

- 1 red onion, cut into quarters and separated by petals

- 2 cups bell peppers, red, green, yellow

- 1 can whole water chestnuts, cut in half

- ½ pound fresh mushrooms, halved

- 32 oz. boneless tuna, chunks or steaks

- 1 Splenda packet

- 2 Zucchini, sliced

- 1 inch thick, keep skins on

Directions

1. Layer the tuna and the vegetable pieces evenly onto 8 skewers.

2. Combine the spices and the oil and chili sauce, add the Splenda

3. Quickly blend, either in a blender or by Quickly whipping.

4. Brush onto the kabob pieces, make sure every piece is coated

5. Grill 4 minutes on each side, check to ensure the tuna is cooked to taste.

6. Serving size is two skewers.

7. Mix the marinade ingredients and store in covered container in the fridge. Place all the vegetables in one container in the fridge.

8. Place the tuna in a separate zip-lock bag.

Nutritional Value: Calories: 467, Total Fat: 18g, Protein: 56g, Total Carbs: 21g, Dietary Fiber: 3.5g, Sugar: 6g, Sodium: 433mg

Salmon with Bok-Choy

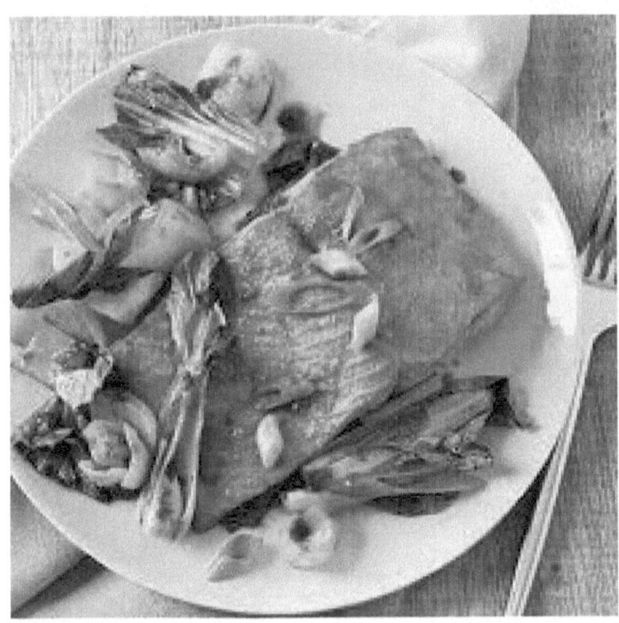

Prep time: 9 minutes

Cook time: 9 minutes

Serves: 4

Ingredients

- 1 cup red peppers, roasted, drained

- 2 cups chopped Bok-Choy

- 1 tablespoon salted butter

- 5 oz. salmon steak

- 1 lemon, sliced very thinly

- ⅛ tablespoon black pepper

- 1 tablespoon olive oil

- 2 tablespoon sriracha sauce

Directions

1. Place oil in skillet

2. Place all but 4 slices of lemon in the skillet.

3. Sprinkle the Bok Choy with the black pepper.

4. Stir fry the Bok-Choy with the lemons.

5. Remove and place on four plates.

6. Place the butter in the skillet and stir fry the salmon, turning once.

7. Place the salmon on the bed of Bok-Choy.

8. Divide the red peppers and encircle the salmon.

9. Place a slice of lemon atop the salmon.

10. Drizzle with sriracha sauce.

11. Freeze the cooked salmon in individual zip-lock bags. Place the Bok-Choy, with the remaining ingredients into one cup containers. Microwave the salmon for one minute and the frozen Bok- Choy for two. Assemble to serve.

Nutritional Value: Calories: 410, Total Fat: 30g, Protein: 30g, Total Carbs: 7g, Dietary Fiber: 2g, Sugar: 0g, Sodium: 200mg

Steak Salad with Asian Spice

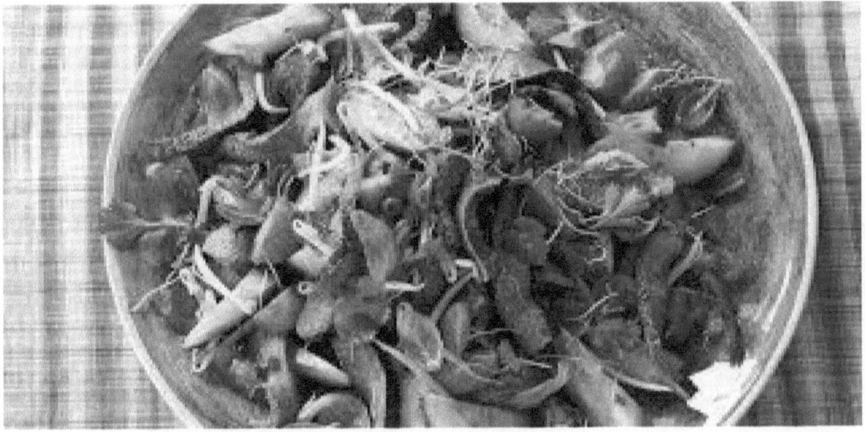

Prep time: 4 minutes

Cook time: 4 minutes

Serves: 2

Ingredients

- 2 tablespoons of sriracha sauce

- 1 tablespoon garlic, minced

- 1 tablespoon ginger, fresh, grated

- 1 bell pepper, yellow, cut into thin strips

- 1 bell pepper, red, cut into thin strips

- 1 tablespoon sesame oil, garlic

- 1 Splenda packet

- ½ tablespoon curry powder

- ½ tablespoon rice wine vinegar

- 8 oz. of beef sirloin, cut into strips

- 2 cups baby spinach, stemmed

- ½ head butter lettuce, torn or chopped into bite-sized pieces

Directions

1. Place the garlic, sriracha sauce, 1 tablespoon sesame oil, rice wine vinegar, and Splenda into a bowl and combine well.

2. Pour half of this mix into a zip-lock bag. Add the steak to marinade while you are preparing the salad.

3. Assemble the brightly colored salad by layering in two bowls.

4. Place the baby spinach into the bottom of the bowl. Place the butter lettuce next.

5. Mix the two peppers and place on top.

6. Remove the steak from the marinade and discard the liquid and bag.

7. Heat the sesame oil and quickly stir fry the steak until desired doneness, it should take about 3 minutes.

8. Place the steak on top of the salad.

9. Drizzle with the remaining dressing (other half of marinade mix).

10. Sprinkle sriracha sauce across the salad.

11. Combine the salad ingredients and place in a zip-lock bag in the fridge. Mix the marinade and halve into 2 zip-lock bags. Place the sriracha sauce into a small sealed container. Slice the steak and freeze in a zip-lock bag with the marinade. To prepare, mix the ingredients like the initial directions. Stir fry the marinated beef for 4 minutes to take into consideration the beef is frozen.

Nutritional Value: Calories: 350, Total Fat: 23g, Protein: 28g, Total Carbs: 7g, Dietary Fiber: 3.5, Sugar: 0, Sodium: 267mg

Parmesan Halibut

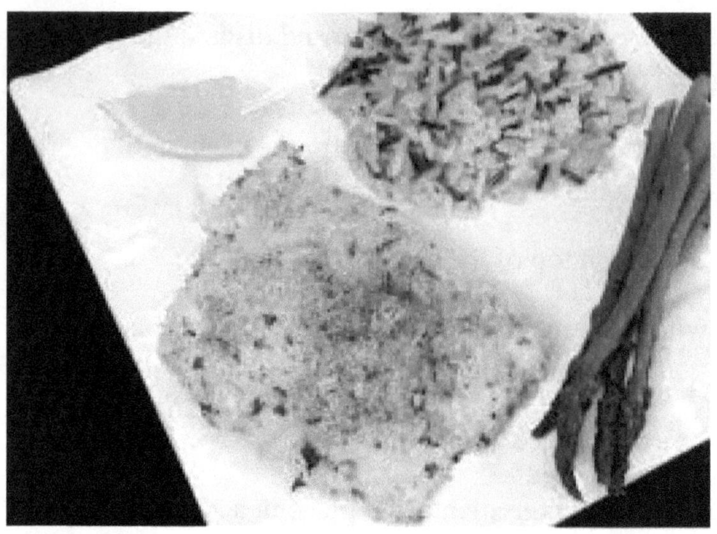

Prep Time: 18 Minutes

Serves: 6

Ingredients:

- 6 halibut fillets

- 1 stick of butter, soft

- 3 tablespoon of parmesan cheese, grated

- 1 tablespoon of panko breadcrumbs, dried

- 1 tablespoon of salt

- ½ tablespoon of black pepper

- 2 tablespoons of garlic powdered, 1 tablespoon of parsley, dried

Directions:

1. Preheat the oven to 400 degrees.

2. Add all the ingredients except for the halibut into a large bowl. Stir well to mix.

3. Pat the halibut fillets dry with a few paper towels and place onto a large baking sheet.

4. Cover each halibut fillet with the parmesan butter mixture.

5. Place into the oven to bake for 10 to 12 minutes.

6. After this time preheat the broiler to high. Broil for 2 to 3 minutes or until golden brown.

7. Remove and serve immediately.

Nutritional Value: Calories: 330, Fat: 30 grams, Carbs: 2 grams, Protein: 13 grams

Keto Friendly Chili

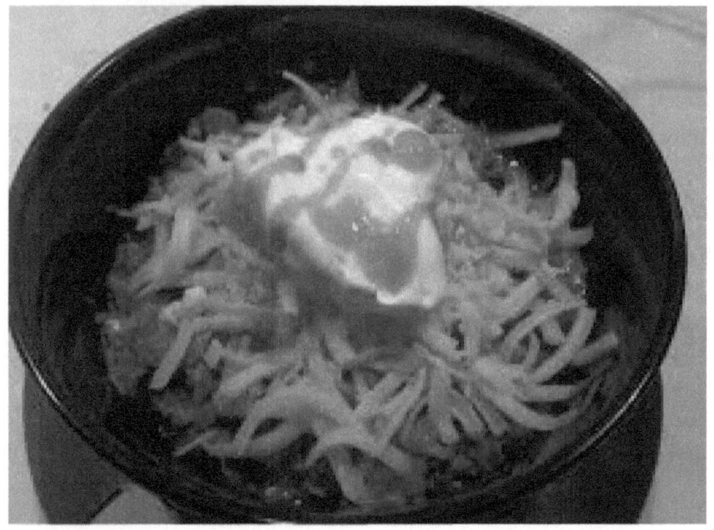

Prep Time: 50 Minutes

Serves: 8

Ingredients:

- 3 tablespoon of extra virgin olive oil

- 1 yellow onion, chopped

- 1 green bell pepper, chopped

- 1 pound of beef, lean and ground

- ½ pound of Italian sausage, ground

- 1 tablespoon of salt

- 1 tablespoon of black pepper

- 2 tablespoons of chili, powdered

- 2 tablespoons of smoked paprika

- 1 tablespoon of cumin, ground

- 1 tablespoon of onion, powdered

- 1 tablespoon of garlic, powdered

- ¼ tablespoon of cayenne 1, 14.5 ounce can of tomatoes, diced

- 1, 6 ounce can of tomato paste

Directions:

1. Place a large soup pot over medium to high heat. Add in the extra virgin olive oil, once the oil is hot enough add in the yellow onion and green bell pepper. Stir well to mix and cook for 3 to 5 minutes or until soft.

2. Add in the beef and Italian sausage. Stir well to mix and cook for 8 to 10 minutes or until the meat is brown.

3. Add in the remaining ingredients and stir well to mix.

4. Bring the mixture to a boil. Once boiling reduce the heat to low and cover. Allow to simmer for 40 minutes.

5. Remove from heat after this time. Serve with a garnish of shredded cheddar cheese and sour cream.

Nutritional Value: Calories: 371, Fat: 31 grams, Carbs: 10 grams, Protein: 13 grams

Tilapia and Broccoli

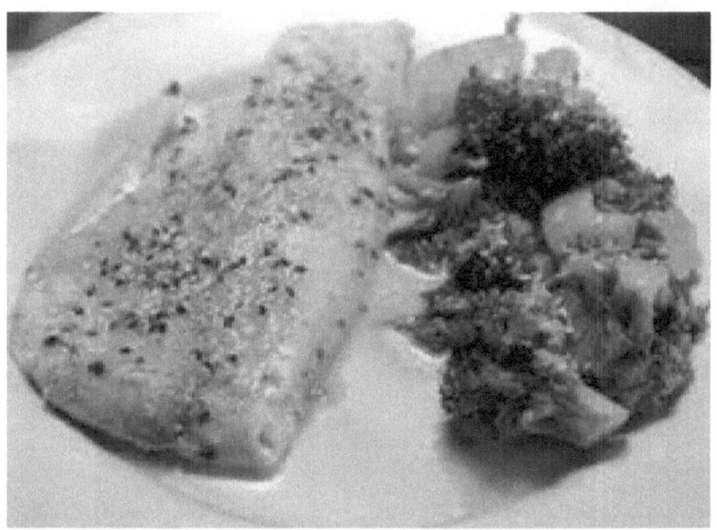

Prep time: 4 minutes

Cook time: 14 minutes

Serves: 1

Ingredients

- 6 oz. tilapia, frozen is fine

- 1 tablespoon butter

- 1 tablespoon garlic, minced or finely chopped

- 1 tablespoon of lemon pepper seasoning

- 1 cup broccoli florets, fresh or frozen, but fresh will be crisper

Directions

1. Set the pre-warmed oven for 350 degrees.

2. Place the fish in an aluminum foil packet.

3. Arrange the broccoli around the fish to make an attractive arrangement.

4. Sprinkle the lemon pepper on the fish.

5. Close the packet and seal, bake for 14 minutes.

6. Combine the garlic and butter. Set aside.

7. Remove the packet from the oven and transfer ingredients to a plate.

8. Place the butter on the fish and broccoli.

9. Place the butter and garlic into small sealed containers or zip-lock bags, Refrigerate or freeze. Cut the broccoli (if fresh) and place in zip-lock bags in the fridge. Place the lemon pepper into a small container.

Nutritional Value: Calories: 362, Total Fat: 25g, Protein: 29g, Total Carbs: 3.5g, Dietary Fiber: 3g, Sugar: 0g, Sodium: 0mg

Hangar Steak

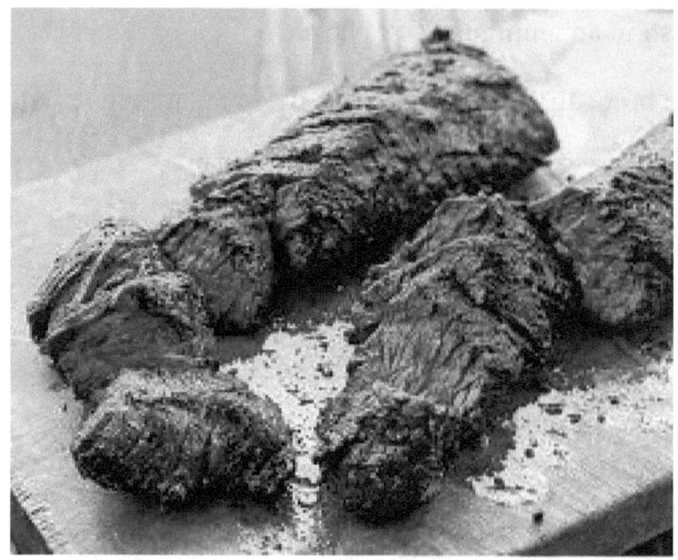

Prep Time: 4 Hours and 15 Minutes

Serves: 8

Ingredients:

- 2 pounds of hanger steak, cleaned and trimmed

- 1 tablespoon of salt

- 1 tablespoon of black pepper

- 1 tablespoon of garlic, granulated

- ½ cup of extra virgin olive

- 2 tablespoon of soy sauce

- 2 tablespoon of vinegar, red wine

- ½ cup of red wine

- 2 tablespoons of rosemary, fresh

- 1 stick of butter, melted

Directions:

1. Add all of the ingredients except for the hangar steak and melted butter into a large bowl. Stir well until evenly mixed.

2. Add in the hangar steak and toss to coat. Cover and set in the fridge to marinate for 4 hours.

3. After this time preheat an outdoor grill to medium heat.

4. Place the marinated steak onto the grill. Grill for 5 to 10 minutes on each side or until cooked to the desired doneness.

5. Remove from the grill and drizzle the melted butter over the steak. Serve.

Nutritional Value: Calories: 338, Fat: 26 grams, Carbs: 1 gram, Protein: 25 grams

Italian Meatballs

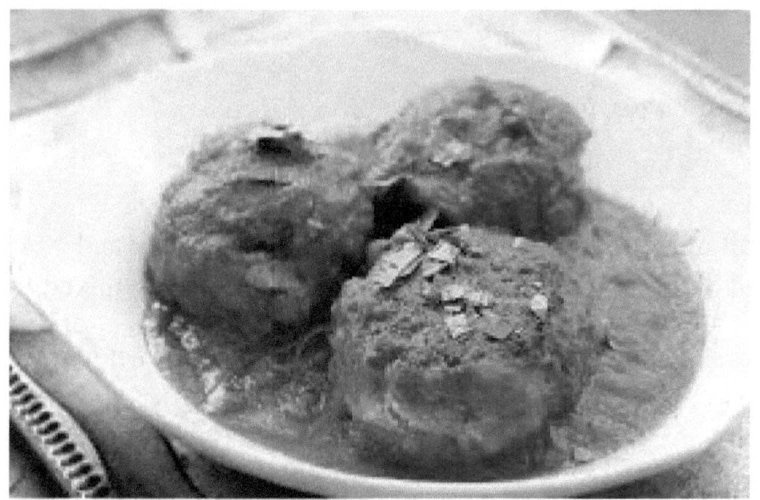

Prep Time: 40 Minutes

Serves: 4

Ingredients:

- 1 pound of beef, lean and ground

- 1 tablespoon of Italian seasoning

- 1 tablespoon of garlic, granulated

- ½ tablespoon of onion, powdered

- 2 tablespoons of salt

- ½ tablespoon of black pepper

- 1 tablespoon of Worcestershire sauce

- 2 tablespoon of tomato paste

- 1 egg, large

- 2 tablespoon of flaxseed meal

- ¼ cup of Parmesan cheese, grated

- ¼ cup of mozzarella cheese, shredded

Directions:

1. Use a large bowl and add in the ground beef, Italian seasoning, garlic, onion, a dash of salt and black pepper, Worcestershire sauce and tomato paste. Stir well to mix.

2. Add the remaining ingredients into the bowl and stir well to mix.

3. Preheat the oven to 400 degrees.

4. While the oven is heating up, form the mixture into even sized meatballs. Place the meatballs onto a lightly greased baking sheet.

5. Place into the oven to bake for 20 minutes or until cooked through.

6. Remove and serve immediately with a meal of your choice.

Nutritional Value: Calories: 451, Fat: 39 grams, Carbs: 3 grams, Protein: 22 grams

Smothered Pan Seared Salmon

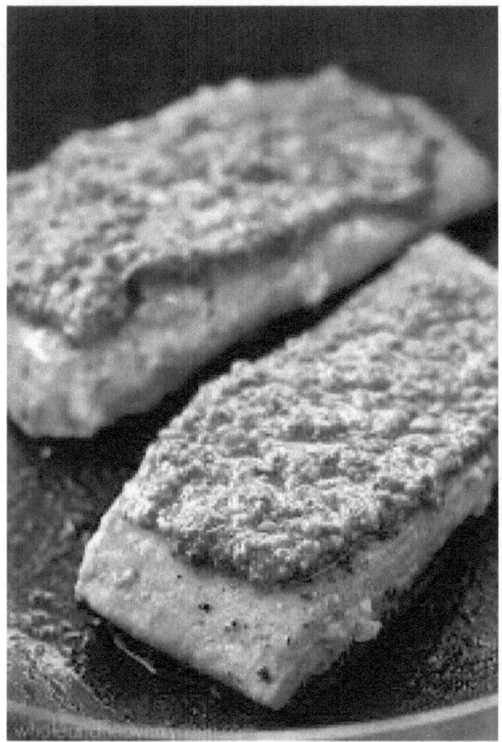

Prep Time: 20 Minutes

Serves: 4

Ingredients:

- 4, 4 ounces salmon fillets

- 2 tablespoons of coconut oil

- 1 Tablespoon of salt

- ½ tablespoon of black pepper

- 1 tablespoon of garlic, powdered

- 1 tablespoon of onion, powdered

- 4 tablespoons of butter

- ½ cup of Greek yogurt, plain

- ½ cup of sour cream

- 2 tablespoon of extra virgin olive

- 1 tablespoon of dill, dried

- 1 lemon, fresh and juice only

- Dash of Tabasco sauce

Directions:

1. Use a medium bowl and add in the salt, black pepper, garlic, and onion. Stir well to mix. Sprinkle this mixture over the salmon fillets. Set the remaining seasoning aside.

2. Place a large skillet over medium to high heat. Add in the coconut oil and once the oil is hot enough add in the salmon fillets. Cook for 3 minutes on each side. Flip and continue to cook for another 3 minutes. Remove and set the salmon aside.

3. Add a tablespoon of butter over each salmon fillet.

4. Add the remaining seasoning, plain yogurt and sour cream into the skillet. Whisk until smooth in consistency. Cook for a further 2 to 3 minutes.

5. Remove from heat and pour the sauce over the top. Serve.

Nutritional Value: Calories: 558, Fat: 58 grams, Carbs: 3 grams, Protein: 24 grams

Healthy Kale Chicken Caesar Salad

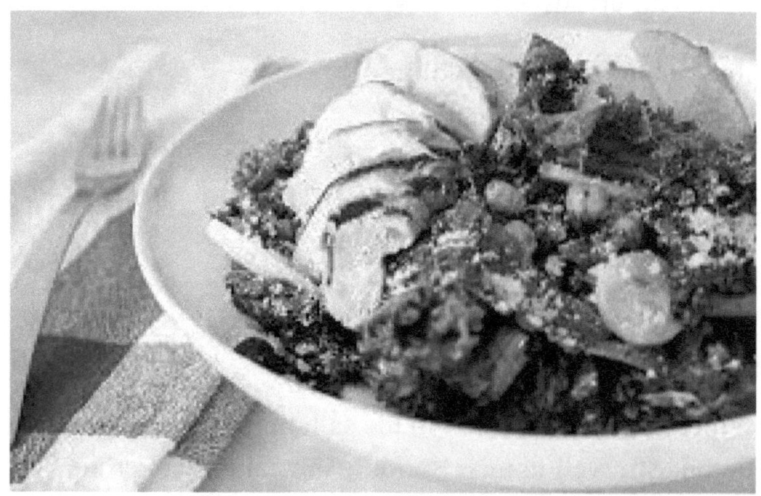

Prep Time: 35 Minutes

Serves: 8

Ingredients for the salad:

- 2 chicken breasts, boneless and skinless

- 4 tablespoon of extra virgin olive oil

- 2 tablespoons of salt

- ½ tablespoon of black pepper

- 1 tablespoon of garlic, powdered

- 1 bunch of kale, washed, chopped and with ribs removed

Ingredients for the salad dressing:

- 1 egg yolk, large

- 2 anchovies

- 1 lemon, fresh and juice only

- 1 tablespoon of apple cider

- ¼ cup of parmesan cheese, grated

- 2 tablespoons of parsley, fresh and chopped

- Dash of salt and black pepper

- ¼ cup of extra virgin olive oil

- 1 to 2 tablespoons of water

Directions:

1. First, preheat the oven to 375 degrees.

2. While the oven is heating up add the chicken breasts into a large bowl. Add in the extra virgin olive oil, dash of salt and black pepper and garlic. Toss well to mix.

3. Place the chicken breasts onto a large baking sheet. Place into the oven to bake for 30 minutes. Remove after this time and slice the chicken into thin strips.

4. Use a food processor and add in all of the ingredients for the salad dressing except for the oil. Blend on the highest setting until smooth in consistency. Then slowly pour in the oil while blending until the dressing is emulsified.

5. Place the kale in a large serving bowl. Add in the chicken and salad dressing. Toss well to mix. Serve immediately.

Nutritional Value: Calories: 208, Fat: 16 grams, Carbs: 8 grams, Protein: 8 grams

Simple Salisbury Steak

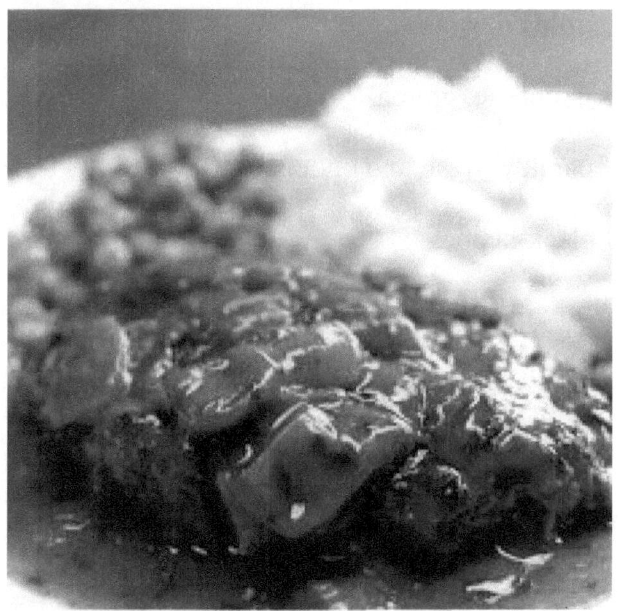

Prep Time: 20 Minutes

Serves: 8

Ingredients for the steak:

- 3 pounds of beef, lean and ground

- ½ cup of panko breadcrumbs

- 2 eggs, large

- 2 tablespoons of ketchup, low in sugar

- 4 tablespoons of mustard, dried

- 8 dashes of Worcestershire sauce

- 1 tablespoon of salt

- 1 tablespoon of black pepper

- 1 tablespoon of garlic, powdered

- 1 tablespoon of onion, powdered

- 2 tablespoons of butter

- 2 tablespoon of extra virgin olive oil

Ingredients for the gravy:

- 1 onion, sliced thinly

- 4 cups of beef broth

- 2 tablespoons of ketchup, low in sugar

- 2 tablespoon of kitchen bouquet

- 8 dashes of Worcestershire sauce

- 2 tablespoons of cornstarch

Directions:

1. Use a large bowl and add in all of the ingredients for the steak except for the butter and extra virgin olive oil. Stir well to mix and form this mixture into patties.

2. Place a large saucepan over medium heat. Add in the extra virgin olive oil and butter. As soon as the butter melts add in the beef patties. Cook for 8 minutes on each side or until cooked through.

3. Remove the cooked patties from the skillet and transfer to a large plate.

4. Add the sliced onions into the skillet. Cook for 5 to 10 minutes or until soft.

5. Then add in the beef broth, low sugar ketchup, kitchen bouquet and Worcestershire sauce. Whisk until smooth in consistency.

6. Add in the cornstarch and whisk to mix. Continue to cook for an additional 2 minutes or until thick in consistency.

7. Add the cooked patties into the gravy and toss to mix.

8. Remove from heat and serve.

Nutritional Value: Calories: 519, Fat: 59 grams, Carbs: 18 grams, Protein: 29 grams

Classic Prime Rib

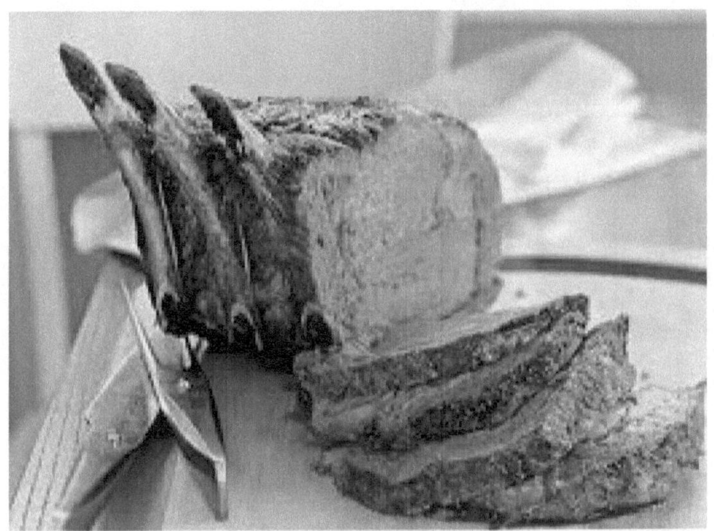

Prep Time: 3 Hours

Serves: 3

Ingredients for the prime rib:

- 1, 8 to 12lbs. prime rib, boneless

- ¼ cup of extra virgin olive oil

- ½ cup of salt

- 1 tablespoon of black pepper

- 2 tablespoons of garlic, granulated

- 1 tablespoon of thyme, dried

- 1 tablespoon of rosemary, dried

- 2 tablespoons of smoked paprika

Ingredients for the horseradish cream:

- 1 cup of sour cream

- ½ cup of mayonnaise

- ¼ cup of horseradish, drained

- ½ of a lemon, juice

- Dash of Tabasco sauce

- Dash of salt and black pepper

Directions:

1. Score the skin of the prime rib with a knife.

2. Drizzle the olive oil over the prime rib. Season with: garlic, thyme, rosemary, paprika and dash of salt and black pepper.

3. Then preheat the oven to 450 to 500 degrees.

4. Place the seasoned prime rib onto a large baking sheet. Place into the oven to roast for 20 minutes. After this time increase the oven to broil and broil for another 8 minutes. Reduce the temperature of the oven to 325 degrees. Roast for 1 hour and 20 minutes.

5. Remove from the oven and set aside to rest for 30 minutes. Slice and serve.

Nutritional Value: Calories: 640, Fat: 56 grams, Carbs: 2 grams, Protein: 33 grams

Zucchini Casserole

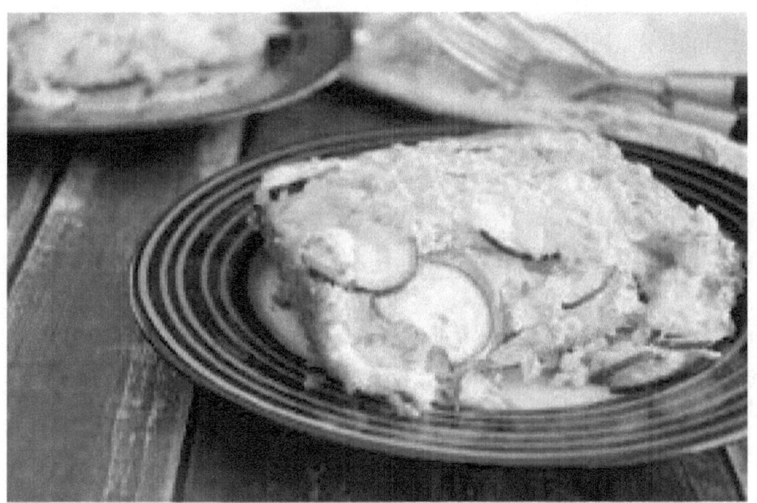

Prep Time: 1 Hour

Serves: 8

Ingredients:

- 5 pieces of bacon, chopped

- 1 onion, chopped

- 2 cloves of garlic, minced

- 2 cups of zucchini, grated

- 1 cup of Colby Jack cheese, grated

- ½ cup of almond flour

- ½ cup of vegetable oil

- ¼ cup of heavy cream

- 6 eggs, large

- Dash of salt and black pepper

Directions:

1. Place a large skillet over low to medium heat. Add in the bacon and cook for 5 minutes or until browned. Transfer the bacon to a large plate lined with paper towels to drain.

2. In the skillet with the bacon fat. Add in the onion and garlic. Stir well to mix and cook for 5 minutes or until soft. Transfer the mixture into a large bowl.

3. Add in the remaining ingredients into the bowl. Whisk well to mix and pour into a large greased baking dish.

4. Top the casserole with the shredded Colby Jack cheese.

5. Place into the oven to bake for 1 hour at 350 degrees. Make sure to turn the casserole after 30 minutes of baking.

6. Remove and allow to cool for 5 minutes before serving.

Nutritional Value: Calories: 334, Fat: 30 grams, Carbs: 6 grams, Protein: 12 grams

Oven Roasted Broccoli with Parmesan Cheese and Garlic

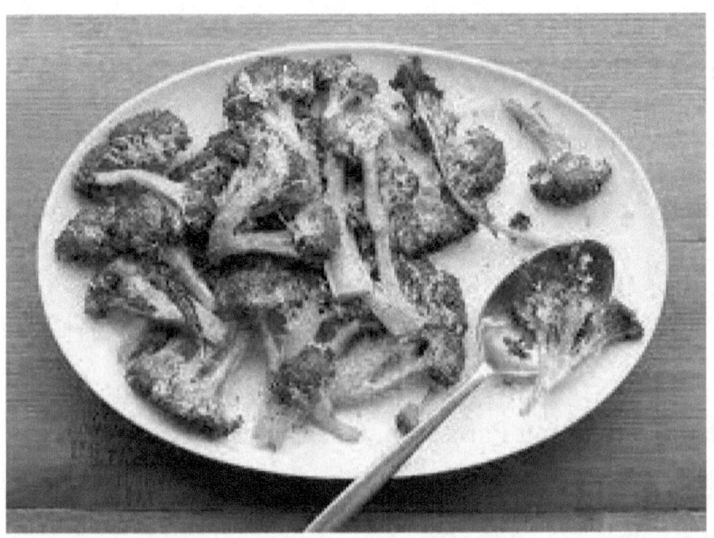

Prep Time: 20 Minutes

Serves: 4

Ingredients:

- 1 head of broccoli, fresh and cut into florets

- 2 cloves of garlic, minced

- ¼ cup of extra virgin olive oil

- Dash of salt and black pepper

- 8 tablespoon of parmesan cheese, grated and divided

- ½ of a lemon, fresh and juice only

Directions:

1. In a medium bowl add in the broccoli florets, garlic, extra virgin olive oil and dash of salt and black pepper.

2. Add in six tablespoons of the grated Parmesan cheese into the mixture and stir well to mix.

3. Add the seasoned broccoli onto a large baking sheet.

4. Place into the oven to roast at 400 degrees for 15 to 20 minutes.

5. Remove from the oven. Squeeze the fresh lemon juice over the top.

6. Sprinkle the remaining Parmesan cheese over the top and toss to coat. Serve.

Nutritional Value: Calories: 242, Fat: 18 grams, Carbs: 11 grams, Protein: 9 grams

Chapter 12: Desserts and Appetizers

Chocolate Truffles

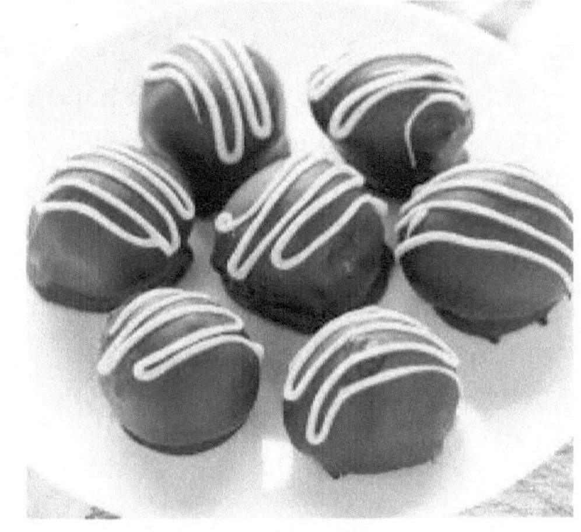

Preparation time: 10 minutes

Cooking time: 6 minutes

Servings: 22

Ingredients:

- 1 cup sugar-free chocolate chips

- 2 tablespoons butter

- ⅔ cup heavy cream

- 2 teaspoons brandy

- 2 tablespoons swerve

- ¼ teaspoon vanilla extract

- Cocoa powder

Directions:

1. Put the heavy cream in a heatproof bowl, add the swerve, butter, and chocolate chips, stir, introduce in a microwave, and heat up for 1 minute.

2. Set aside for 5 minutes, stir well, and mix with brandy, and vanilla extract.

3. Stir again and set aside in the refrigerator for a couple of hours.

4. Use a melon baller to shape the truffles, roll them in cocoa powder, and serve.

Nutritional Value: Calories - 60, Fat - 5, Fiber - 4, Carbs - 6, Protein - 1

Doughnuts

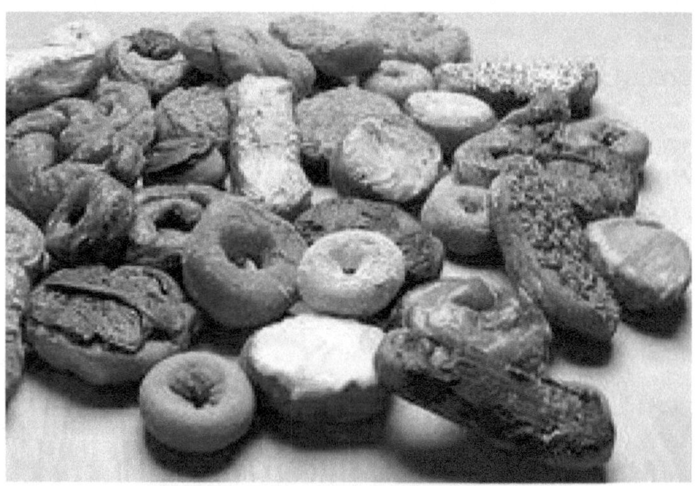

Preparation time: 10 minutes

Cooking time: 15 minutes

Servings: 24

Ingredients:

- ¼ cup erythritol

- ¼ cup flaxseed meal

- ¾ cup almond flour

- 1 teaspoon baking powder

- 1 teaspoon vanilla extract

- 2 eggs

- 3 tablespoons coconut oil

- ¼ cup coconut milk

- 20 drops red food coloring

- A pinch of salt

- 1 tablespoon cocoa powder

Directions:

1. In a bowl, mix the flaxseed meal with almond flour, cocoa powder, baking powder, erythritol, and salt, and stir.

2. In another bowl, mix the coconut oil with coconut milk, vanilla extract, food coloring, and eggs, and stir.

3. Combine the 2 mixtures, stir using a hand mixer, transfer to a bag, make a hole in the bag, and shape 12 doughnuts on a baking sheet.

4. Place in an oven at 350°F and bake for 15 minutes. Arrange them on a platter and serve.

Nutritional Value: Calories - 60, Fat - 4, Fiber - 0, Carbs - 1, Protein - 2

Chocolate Bombs

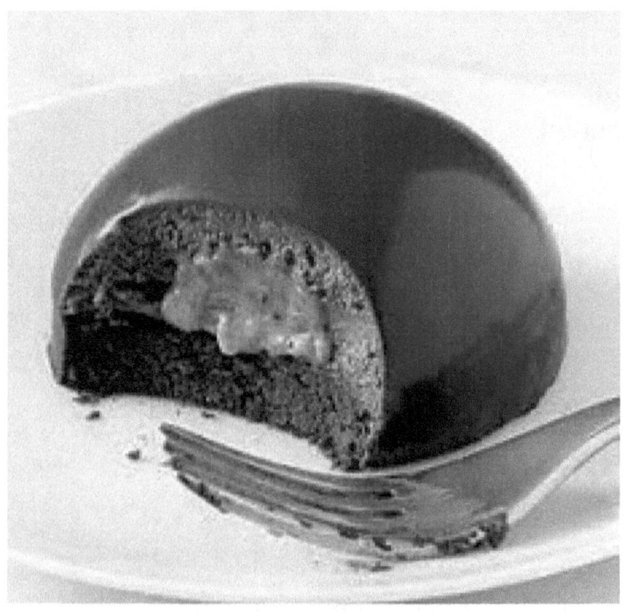

Preparation time: 10 minutes

Cooking time: 10 minutes

Servings: 12

Ingredients:

- 10 tablespoons coconut oil

- 3 tablespoons macadamia nuts, chopped

- 2 packets stevia

- 5 tablespoons unsweetened coconut powder

- A pinch of salt

Directions:

1. Put the coconut oil in a pot and melt over medium heat.

2. Add the stevia, salt, and cocoa powder, stir well, and take off the heat. Spoon this into a candy tray and keep in the refrigerator for a couple of hours.

3. Sprinkle the macadamia nuts on top and keep in the refrigerator until ready to serve.

Nutritional Value: Calories - 50, Fat - 1, Fiber - 0, Carbs - 1, Protein - 2

Kale Crackers

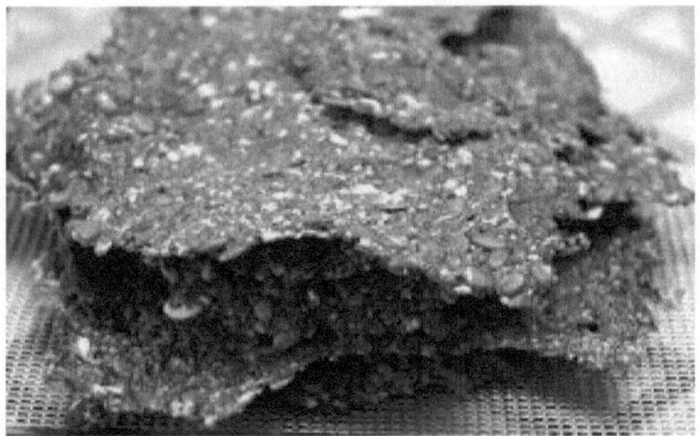

Ingredients

- 3 tablespoons Filtered Water

- ½ cup Fresh Kale, trimmed and chopped

- ½ cup, plus 2 tablespoons, Whole Wheat Flour

- ½ teaspoon Dried Rosemary, crushed

- Pinch of Himalayan Pink Salt

- Pinch of Red Pepper Flakes, crushed

- 2 tablespoons Almond Butter

Directions

1.   Preheat the oven to 400 degrees F and line a large baking sheet with parchment paper.

2.   In a blender, add the water and kale and pulse until smooth. In a bowl, mix the flour, rosemary, salt and red pepper flakes. Add the butter and mix until the mixture becomes crumbly. Stir in the kale mixture and mix until dough forms. Roll the dough into a thin layer on a floured smooth surface. Cut the rolled dough according to your desired shape.

3.   Carefully place the crackers onto the prepared baking sheet and bake for 8 to 10 minutes.

Bean Bruschetta

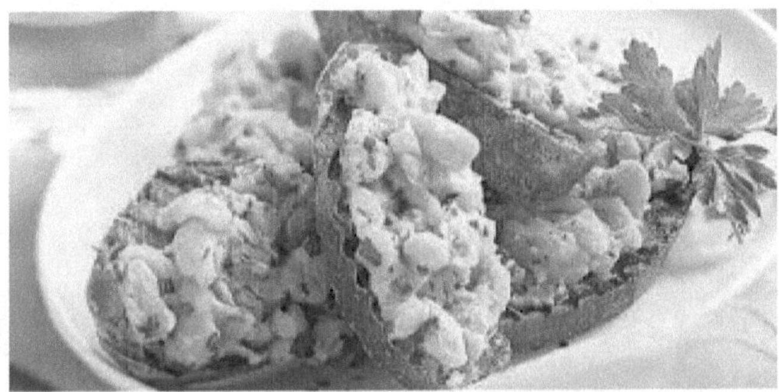

Ingredients

- ¾ cup cooked White Beans

- 1 medium Tomato, chopped

- ½ Garlic Clove, minced

- 2 tablespoons Fresh Scallion, chopped

- 1 tablespoon Balsamic Vinegar

- ⅛ teaspoon Red Pepper Flakes, crushed

- Pinch of Himalayan Pink Salt

- 8 (½-inch thick) toasted Whole Wheat Bread Slices

Directions

1. In a bowl, except for the bread slices, mix all of the ingredients.

2. Place the bean mixture over the bread slices and serve immediately.

Fruit Kabobs with Dip

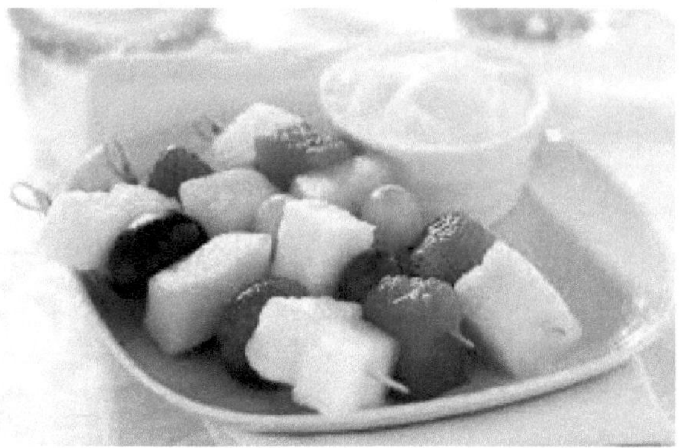

Ingredients

For Dip:

- 1 cup Raw Cashew nuts, soaked overnight and drained

- ½ cup Fresh Cherries, pitted

- ⅓ cup Almond Milk, unsweetened

- 1 tablespoon Pure Maple Syrup

- 1 teaspoon Vanilla Extract

For Kabobs:

- 1 Orange, peeled, seeded and sectioned

- 1 Apple, peeled, cored and cubed

- 1 Kiwi, peeled and cubed

- 2 Bananas, peeled and sliced

- 6-8 Strawberries, hulled and sliced

- ¼ cup Raspberries

Directions

1.   For dip, add all of the ingredients into a blender and pulse until smooth. Transfer the dip to a bowl. Cover and refrigerate for 6 to 8 hours.

2.   Thread the fruit pieces onto skewers according to your preference. Serve with the chilled dip.

Grilled Vegetable Kabobs

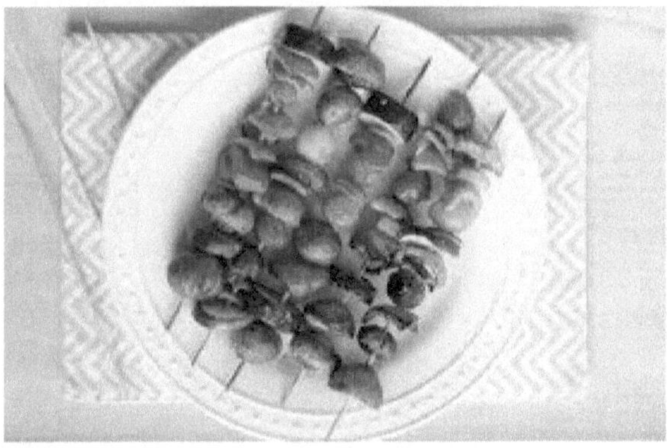

Ingredients

For Vegetable Kabobs:

- 2 Yellow Squash, sliced into 1-inch pieces

- 2 Zucchinis, sliced into 1-inch pieces

- 1 Red Bell Pepper, seeded and cut into chunks

- 1 Green Bell Pepper, seeded and cut into chunks

- ½ pound Fresh Mushrooms

- 12 Cherry Tomatoes

- 1 Red Onion, cut into chunks

- 2 tablespoons Almond Butter

For Dressing:

- ½ cup Avocado, peeled, pitted and chopped

- 1 small Garlic Clove, chopped

- ¼ cup Fresh Chives

- 2 tablespoons Fresh Basil Leaves

- 3 tablespoons Fresh Lemon juice

- ¼ cup Almond Butter

- Pinch of Himalayan Pink Salt

- Freshly Ground Black Pepper, as required

Directions:

1.   Preheat the grill to medium heat.

2.   Thread the vegetables onto the pre-soaked wooden skewers and evenly coat with the almond butter. Grill for about 15 minutes, turning after every 5 minutes.

3.   Meanwhile, add all of the dressing ingredients into a food processor and pulse until smooth. Serve the vegetable kabobs with the dressing.

Colorful Berry Salad

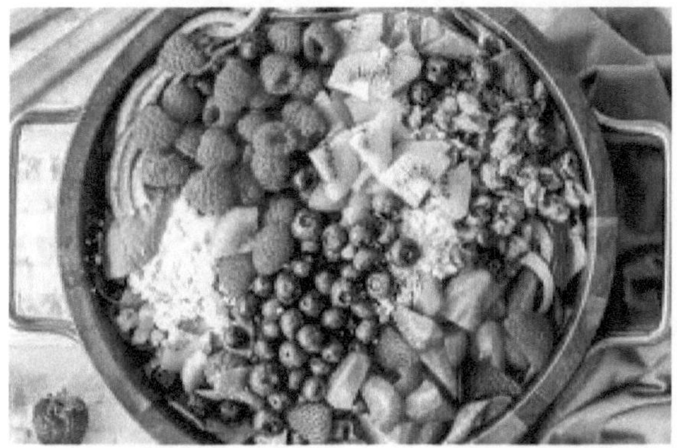

Ingredients

- 1 cup Fresh Strawberries

- 1 cup Fresh Raspberries

- ¾ cup Fresh Blueberries

- ¾ cup Fresh Blackberries

- ¼ cup Fresh Cranberries

- 1 tablespoon Fresh Lime juice

- ½ tablespoon Pure Maple Syrup

- ¼ cup Almonds, toasted and chopped

- 1 tablespoon Mint Leaves, freshly chopped

Directions

1. In a large serving bowl, mix all of the berries.

2. Add the lime juice and maple syrup and toss to coat.

3. Garnish with the almonds and mint leaves before serving.

Strawberry Spinach Salad

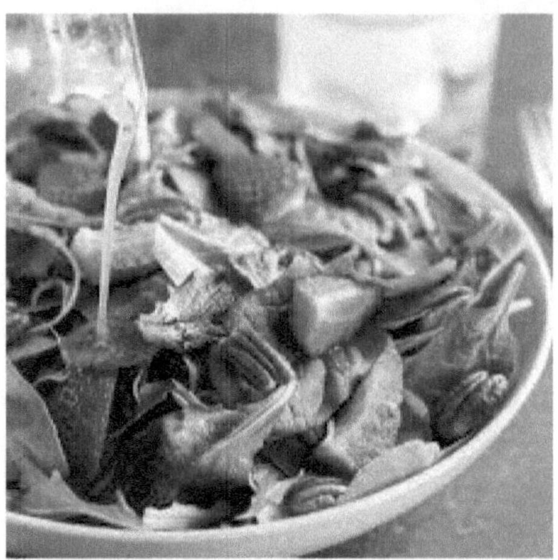

Ingredients

For Vinaigrette:

- 1 small Garlic Clove, minced

- ¼ teaspoon Fresh Dill Weed

- ½ tablespoon Apple Cider Vinegar

- 1 tablespoon Fresh Lime juice

- 1 tablespoon Pure Maple Syrup

- Pinch of Freshly Ground Black Pepper

For Salad

- 1 cup Fresh Strawberries, hulled and sliced

- 4 cups Fresh Baby Spinach

- 1 Scallion, chopped

- 1 tablespoon Walnuts, chopped

Directions

1.   In a small bowl, mix the garlic, dill weed, vinegar, lime juice, maple syrup and black pepper.

2.   In a large salad bowl, mix the strawberries, spinach, and scallion. Pour the vinaigrette over the salad and toss to coat well. Top with the walnuts and serve.

Apple & Pear Salad

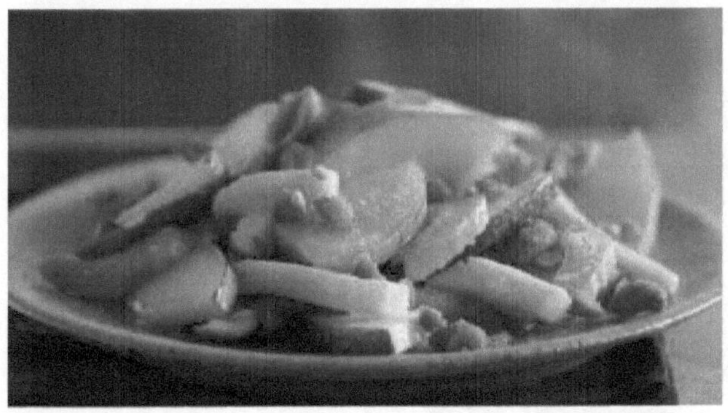

Ingredients

For Strawberry Vinaigrette:

- ½ cup Fresh Strawberries, hulled and sliced

- 2 large Medjool Dates, pitted and chopped

- 2 tablespoons Pecans, chopped

- ¼ cup Filtered Water

- ¼ cup Fresh Orange juice

- 1 tablespoon Apple Cider Vinegar

For Salad

- 1 large Apple, peeled, cored and sliced

- 1 large Pear, peeled, cored and sliced

- 4 cups Fresh Mixed Greens

- 2 tablespoons Pumpkin Seeds, toasted

Directions

1. In a blender, add all the vinaigrette ingredients and pulse until smooth.

2. In a large salad bowl, mix the fruits and greens. Pour the vinaigrette over the salad and toss to coat well. Top with the pumpkin seeds and serve.

Mixed Citrus Salad

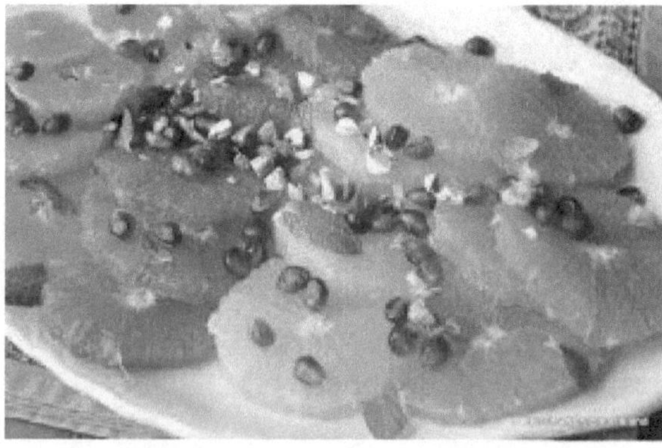

Ingredients

- 1 Naval Orange, peeled, seeded and sectioned

- 1 Mandarin Orange, peeled, seeded and sectioned

- 2 Grape Fruits, peeled, seeded and sectioned

- ½ tablespoon Pure Maple Syrup

- 1 tablespoon Mint Leaves, freshly chopped

- 1 teaspoon Orange Zest, freshly grated

Directions

1.   In a large serving bowl, mix all the ingredients, except for the orange zest. Cover and refrigerate to chill before serving.

2.   Garnish with the orange zest and serve.

Chapter 13: Soups and Stews

Bok-Choy Ginger Soup

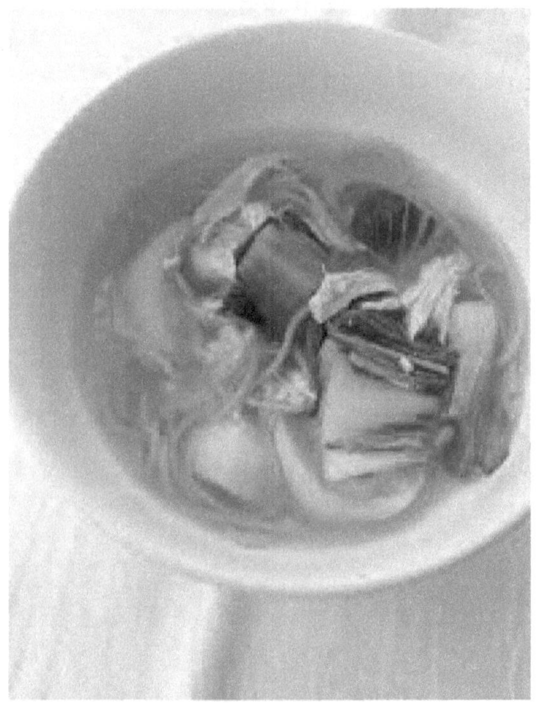

Prep time: 9 minutes

Cook time: 9 minutes

Serves: 4

Ingredients

- 3 cups diced green onions

- 2 cups chopped or sliced mushrooms

- 3 tablespoon fresh grated ginger

- 3 tablespoon minced garlic

- 4 T tamari

- 2 cups chopped Bok-Choy

- 1 T Cilantro, chopped

- 6 oz. firm tofu, cut into bite sized squares

- 3 T grated carrot

- 1 can diced tomatoes and peppers

- 6 cups chicken broth

Directions

1. Place everything but the green onions, tofu, and carrot into a sauce and bring to a boil.

2. Reduce the heat to low-med and cook this for 6 minutes.

3. Stir in the green onions, tofu, and carrots. Cook for 2 more minutes.

4. Serve sprinkled with the cilantro.

Nutritional Value: Calories: 65, Total Fat: 2g, Protein: 7g, Total Carbs: 5g, Dietary Fiber: 2g, Sugar: 0g, Sodium: 100mg

Cream of Mushroom Soup

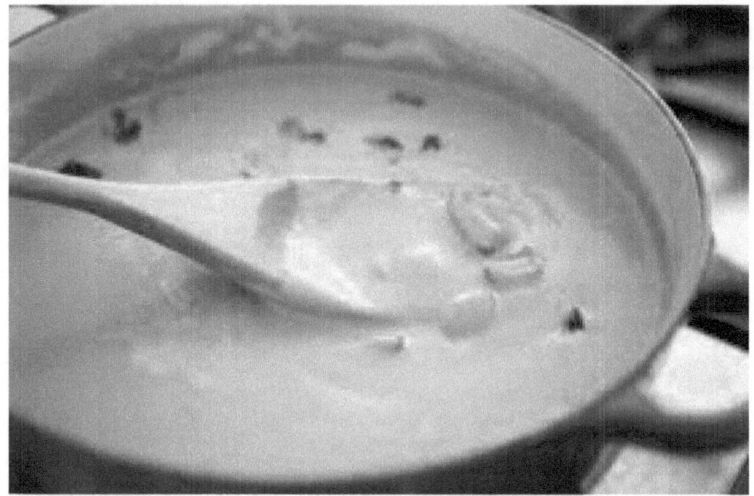

Prep time: 6 minutes

Cook time: 4 minutes

Serves: 4

Ingredients

- 1 pound of mushrooms, sliced

- 1 T butter

- ¼ cup cream

- 1 cup water

- ¼ grated Parmesan cheese

- dash of basil

- dash of black pepper

Directions

1. Microwave the mushrooms in the water for 4 minutes. Taste for the desired doneness.

2. Drain the mushrooms.

3. Place in blender with butter and cream and Parmesan.

4. Blend until creamy.

5. Pour into bowl and serve

Nutritional Value: Calories: 210, Total Fat: 17g, Protein: 10g, Total Carbs: 3g, Dietary Fiber: 0.5g, Sugar: 0g, Sodium: 370mg

Cucumber Soup

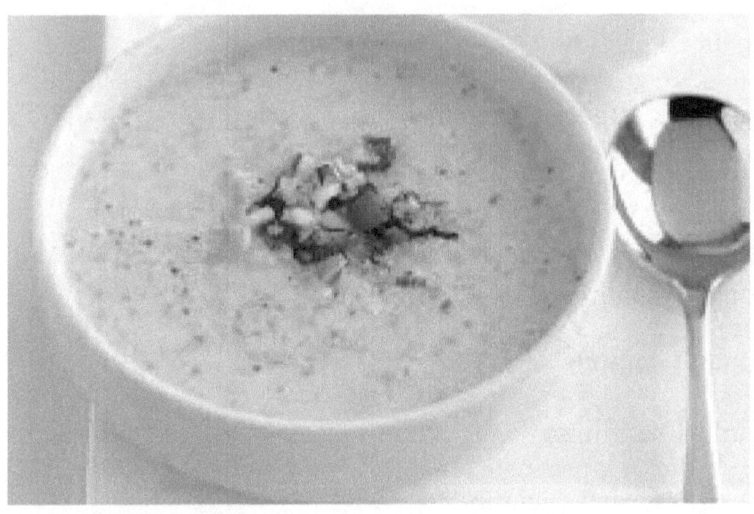

Prep time: 14 minutes

Cook time: none

Serves: 4

Ingredients

- 2 T minced garlic

- 4 c English cucumbers, peeled and diced

- ½ c onion, diced

- 1 T lemon juice

- 1 ½ cups chicken broth

- ½ tablespoon salt

- 1 diced avocado

- ¼ tablespoon red pepper flakes

- ¼ cup diced parsley

- ½ cup Greek yogurt, plain

Directions

1. Place all the ingredients and emulsify by blending, except ½ c chopped cucumber.

2. Blend until smooth.

3. Pour into 4 servings.

4. Top with reserved cucumber.

5. Freeze in one cup containers with lids. Let thaw to serve or microwave 2 minutes to serve hot.

Nutritional Value: Calories: 169, Total Fat: 12g, Protein: 4g, Total Carbs: 9g, Dietary Fiber: 5g, Sugar: 6g, Sodium: 494mg

Cauliflower Soup

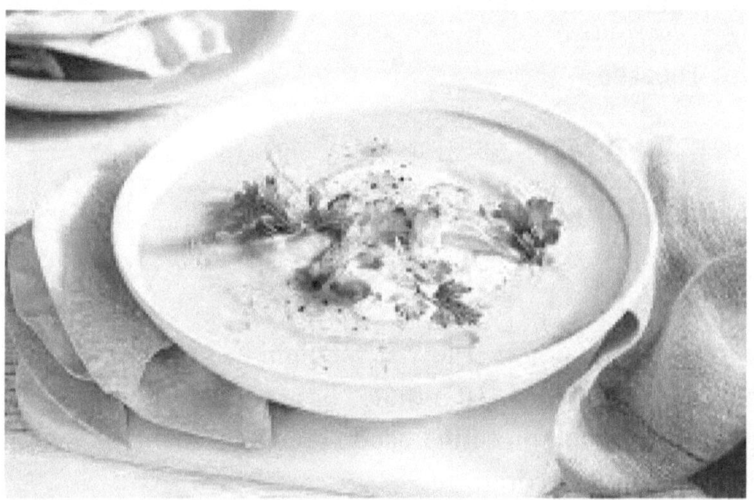

Prep Time: 1 Hour and 45 Minutes

Serves: 4

Ingredients:

- 1 head of cauliflower, fresh

- 6 pieces of bacon, chopped

- 3 tablespoons of butter

- 1 onion, chopped

- 2 cloves of garlic, minced

- 2 tablespoons of thyme, fresh

- 3 cups of chicken stock

- 2 cups of heavy cream

- ½ cup of Parmesan cheese, grated

- Dash of salt and black pepper

- Dash of Tabasco

- ½ tablespoon of lemon juice, fresh

- 1 tablespoon of chives, chopped

Directions:

1. Place a large soup pot over low to medium heat. Add in the bacon and cook for 8 to 10 minutes or until the bacon is crispy. Remove and place the bacon onto a large plate lined with paper towels to drain.

2. Add in the butter and once the butter is melted add in the onion and garlic. Stir to mix and cook for 5 minutes or until the onion is soft.

3. Add in the fresh cauliflower, thyme and chicken stock. Stir well to mix.

4. Bring the mixture to a boil. Once boiling reduce the heat to low and add in the heavy cream. Stir well to incorporate. Cover and cook for 15 to 20 minutes or until the cauliflower is soft.

5. Remove the soup pot from heat. Pour the soup into a blender. Blend on the highest setting until smooth in consistency.

6. Pour the soup back into the pot and place back over low to medium heat.

7. Add in the fresh lemon juice, Parmesan cheese and Tabasco sauce. Whisk to mix.

8. Season with a dash of salt and black pepper.

9. Remove from heat and serve the soup with a topping of bacon and a sprinkling of chives.

Nutritional Value: Calories: 686, Fat: 62 grams, Carbs: 14 grams, Protein: 18 grams

Conclusion

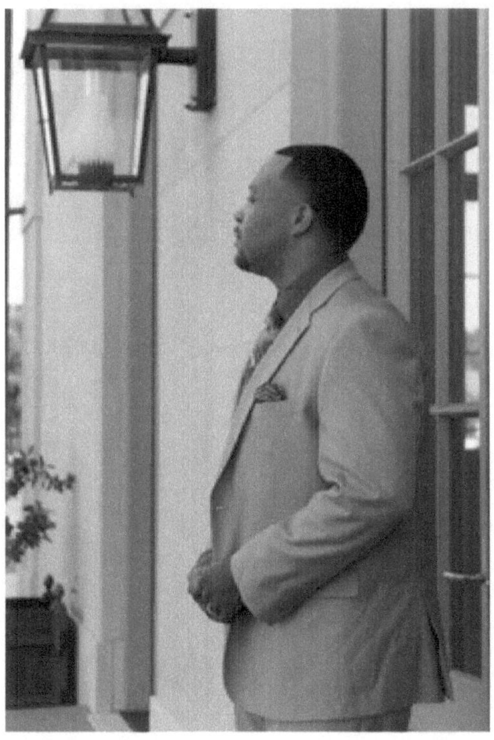

There you have it – the "Thinker's Diet" also known as the Keto Diet. At this point, you already know what it is, why it's good for you, how to implement or introduce the "Thinker's Diet", and how to tell if you've already reached a state of ketosis. You also have sample meal plans and tips for staying "Thinking" while eating out, and delicious recipes to try at home. You now know enough about the "Thinker's Diet" to start enjoying its benefits.

The "Thinker's Diet" is a great way to watch pounds melt away, quickly and safely. Your own body turns into a fat burning machine, using up stores of fat rather than glucose from the food you're eating for energy.

At the same time, it protects your heart and other muscles from damage since you're feeding them nourishing, healthy oils and lots of needed protein.

For the "Thinker's Diet" to work, you don't need to count calories and weigh or measure your food necessarily, but as with all eating plans, you need to be honest with yourself about what you're eating and how much.

I want you to remember though, no matter how much you try to lose that extra body fat, you must take your age into consideration. Especially if you have already passed middle age, you need to accept that you can no longer have the body you had when you were 20 or 30. Sometimes, in the quest to be our best, we may forget that we have a wholesome, working body – far more than a lot of people can say.

But don't lose heart, while the time to look your "best" may have passed, the time to just shed a few pounds, enjoy your body and live a healthier life is now! Try your best to find a balance between living healthily and being happy with the body you have. Make sure to follow this simple cookbook guide to help you lose weight and live an overall healthier lifestyle. So, what are you waiting for – get slow cooking!

While virtually unlimited fats are allowed, it's good to get healthy, unsaturated fats that your body can easily digest, and which won't clog your arteries; this means fats from fish, avocados, and peanuts, and olive oil. Lean protein choices are also better than fatty cuts of beef.

As with the rest of your food, you don't necessarily need to count carbohydrates, as long as you educate yourself about which foods are high in carbs and are sure to limit these in your diet.

If you do follow the ketogenic diet as recommended, you'll get a lean and toned physique in no time. You'll also calm your cravings, have a consistent source of energy, and won't feel fatigued throughout the day as you usually would.

The next step is to take the necessary action and put into practice what you have learned. Don't forget to consult your doctor before you start any kind of diet, especially if you have some underlying condition. All in all, I hope you enjoyed the book!

I'd like to give a special thanks to my beautiful wife Mrs. Crystal N. Dugar who always loved me unconditionally. Thank you to my photographer Erica Butler, she can be reached at www.instagram.com/e.r.b_photography_. I thank God for Devante Blackwell CEO of "Captivating Cinema" from Lake Charles, LA for being a good friend to me and for filming all my video footage. He can be reached at www.captivatingcinema.com. I'd also like to thank my friend/personal trainer Beau Richard CEO of "Team Fit" in Lake Charles, LA for allowing God to use him to help me get on the right track and always having a word of encouragement. Lastly, I want to think my best friend Jeremy Shelton CEO of "Kingdom Kuttz" in Lake Charles, LA for being a true friend. I thank God for you PREEEACH!

Remember, you can do ALL things through Christ, and ONLY what you do for Christ will last. God Bless You.

-- [Marlon J. Dugar]

www.ingramcontent.com/pod-product-compliance
Lightning Source LLC
Chambersburg PA
CBHW031229250726
48655CB00005B/1872